Migraine Headaches.

Managing Migraines.

How to effectively cope with migraines: migraine pain relief, treatment and natural remedies.

by

Robert Rymore

ALL RIGHTS RESERVED. This book contains material protected under International and Federal Copyright Laws and Treaties.

Any unauthorized reprint or use of this material is strictly prohibited. No part of this book may be reproduced or transmitted in any form or by any means, electronic, mechanical or otherwise, including photocopying or recording, or by any information storage and retrieval system without express written permission from the author.

Copyrighted © 2014

Published by: IMB Publishing

Acknowledgements

Special Thanks to Harvey B. for writing the diet plans.
Thank you to Tim Allardyce from Croydon Physio
Marilyn Devonish from Trance Formations
Paul Knowles
Tamzin Freeman

And the staff at the Acumedic Clinic for their explanations of Chinese Medicine and Acupuncture.
Acumedic can be found at: 101-105 Camden High Street, NW1 7JN.
The contact number is +44(0)20 7388 6704, the main website is www.acumedic.com.

Table of Contents

Acknowledgements 3

Statistics and Facts 5

Introduction 6

Chapter 1) Migraines 7

Chapter 2) Medications and Treatments for Migraines 16

Chapter 3) Treating Migraines Naturally 27

Chapter 4) Food Triggers, Diet and Nutrition 41

Chapter 5) The Hormone Link 47

Chapter 6) Other Causes of Head Pain 58

Chapter 7) Coping With a Migraine 62

Chapter 8) Stress Relief 70

Chapter 9) Blood Sugar Control 81

Chapter 10) Stretching, Yoga and Meditation 87

Chapter 11) Recipes 99

Appendix One: Migraines, A Personal Experience 118

Appendix Two: Stress Relieving Advice 120

Resources 122

Further Reading 124

Statistics and Facts

Currently, there is no cure for migraine sufferers, however, there are many medications that can help to effectively treat and manage the condition.

Migraines can often begin during puberty and adults aged 35-45 are the most commonly affected.

Migraines have a significant effect on people's lives, affecting their ability to work and their productivity. Figures from the World Health Organization show that migraines cost 25 million working or school days every year. Migraines can also be severe enough to be a constant source of disability.

WHO has also questioned the amount of effective care that is received by migraine patients. Statistics show that only half of the people in the United States and United Kingdom suffering from migraines had seen a doctor in the past 12 months and two thirds of patients had been misdiagnosed; many patients depend on over-the-counter medication for their migraines and do not get any other help.

Introduction

Migraines are a painful and distressing condition that blights the lives of sufferers.

The aim of this book is to explain the many different treatments that are available to sufferers as well as to share other people's personal experience of migraines and the tips and tricks that they use to help manage their migraines.

The book will begin by explaining what a migraine is and detail the symptoms that are experienced by sufferers. The various triggers for migraines will be discussed as well as the different treatments – both medical and natural – will also be detailed.

Later on in the book there are also detailed chapters on practical tips that the reader can use to help address the causes of their migraines. Whether stress or hormones are a factor, the reader will find chapters on how to better manage these issues.

By learning more about migraines, their causes, and the steps that can be taken to better manage the condition, the reader can gain some control over their lives by taking the necessary steps to reduce the chances of a migraine and learn about the various methods that are available to treat and manage the migraines more effectively. As ever, before using an alternative remedy, it is important to discuss any therapies or natural treatments with a physician as some of the therapies might interact with medication that the patient is already on.

In addition, it isn't a good idea to radically change the diet, or to drastically alter the daily routine, as both of these factors can make the occurrence of migraines worse, especially if they are induced by low blood sugar or if they are stress-related, so it is important to seek advice before making any major changes to diet or lifestyle.

Chapter 1) Migraines

1) What is a migraine?
Patients suffering from a migraine will experience a severe headache, often with other symptoms that will precede the headache. The pain is intense and can even leave some grown adults in tears; such is the severity of it.

The pain will often be described as a throbbing pain and it can last for several days at a time. The pain from migraine is usually felt on one side of the head; however, the pain can sometimes be bi-lateral.

Migraines are often considered as neurological; however, recent research suggests that the cause might be vascular.

Patients can also experience sensory symptoms such as tingling and some suffer problems with their speech during a migraine attack.

As detailed below migraines are often divided into two different groups:

Episodic Migraines:
If a patient has migraines for less than 15 days of the month, then these would be classed as episodic migraines.

Chronic migraines:
Patients experiencing chronic migraines get them for 15 days of the month or more.

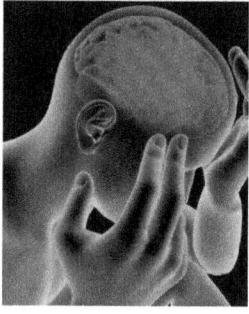

Chapter 1) Migraines

2) Different types of Migraine

a) Migraine with aura

Patients who experience a migraine with aura will experience a visual disturbance before an attack. The visual disturbances will be different for each person but common symptoms include a zig zag pattern in front of the eyes, flashing lights, spots, lines in front, etc. Sometimes the visual disturbances will vary before each attack so prior to a migraine a patient might experience flashing lights, while on another occasion they might have a zig zag pattern.

Diagnosis

No tests are usually needed to diagnose a migraine and they will usually be diagnosed by your GP/physician. Further tests won't normally be deemed necessary, however, if the migraines become more severe or more frequent then the patient will usually be referred to a neurologist for further tests to see if there is an underlying cause for the migraines.

Symptoms

Other symptoms of a migraine include nausea and vomiting, sensitivity to light and sound. The patient might also have problems concentrating both before and after the migraine and they might also experience problems with memory during or after an attack. Some patients might also feel dizzy and others find that their balance and co-ordination is a problem. If the nausea is bad, then patients will often find it difficult to eat or find that they don't feel like food.

Migraines can last for a few hours and sometimes they can last for days.

After a migraine, a patient can feel weak and tired and resting until the migraine is completely over is often the only option.

b) Migraine without aura

Patients who experience migraines without aura do not get the visual disturbances prior to an attack, they do, however, get all of the other symptoms that a typical migraine sufferer will get. These types of migraines can sometimes be little bit more difficult to manage, as there aren't always any warning signs of a migraine attack, however, if a patient has had migraines for a while then they will have learned to recognise the other signs and symptoms of a migraine coming on.

Symptoms:

Common symptoms of these types of migraine include nausea, vomiting, sensitivity to light and sound, and feelings of tiredness prior to the attack.

Diagnosis:

Again, these types of migraines will be diagnosed by a doctor/physician and further tests won't usually be considered necessary unless the migraines get worse.

c) Silent Migraines

Silent migraines can prove to be a major medical issue for some people and, if severe, they can interfere with everyday life. Patients with silent migraines get all of the other symptoms of a migraine such as nausea, sensitivity to light and an aura that will cause visual disturbances, however, they won't get the actual migraine.

Some patients can go for years experiencing these kinds of symptoms without fully understanding what is happening and other patients can live in fear of a migraine attack as they have all of the symptoms of one, but the migraine doesn't occur.

Diagnosis:

These types of migraines can sometimes be difficult to diagnose due to the vague symptoms. If it is suspected that there is an underlying condition causing the symptoms then a referral will usually be made to a neurologist.

d) Ocular Migraines
An ocular migraine is much rarer than other types of migraine. An ocular migraine, sometimes called a retinal migraine, occurs in the occipital cortex of the brain. This part of the brain influences the vision and the most common symptoms of this type of migraine is a visual disturbance.

In patients with ocular migraines, just one eye will be affected. Some patients with ocular migraines have a blind spot in their eye during the migraine while other patients can't see out of the affected eye at all. Once the migraine has subsided, the eyesight will return to normal.

These types of migraines can occur without any other signs or symptoms, which is quite common, or they might be coupled with the typical symptoms of a migraine.
Ocular migraines can last from twenty minutes- two hours, but the pain can be difficult to manage when they occur and the visual disturbances can be frightening for patients, especially when they first start to experience the symptoms.
Some patients can experience several attacks in one day and some people report repeated attacks over the course of a week.

Symptoms of an Ocular migraine

The symptoms of an ocular migraine are often the same as a regular migraine. Ocular migraines begin with visual disturbances; these symptoms can include flashing lights, zig zags and spots in front of the eyes.
During the attack some patients will also experience symptoms such as nausea, vomiting, sensitivity to light and sensitivity to sound.

Chapter 1) Migraines

Diagnosis of ocular migraines

A doctor/physician will usually diagnose ocular migraines once the patient has described the symptoms and detailed how often the attacks are. There isn't usually a need for further tests; however, if the symptoms are severe and frequent then the patient might be referred to a neurologist and further tests will be carried out to see if there is an underlying cause.

e) Abdominal Migraines
These types of migraines tend to affect children, but can also affect adults. Symptoms include stomach pain, which can last up to three days, feelings of sickness and lack of appetite.

3) Famous Sufferers
It is believed that up to one in ten people suffer from migraines – and this includes celebrities. Famous sufferers include Elvis Presley, Julius Caesar, Charles Darwin, Napoleon Bonaparte, and writer Virginia Woolf are just some of the famous people that suffer from migraines. Migraines are also common among creative people such as artists.

4) Migraine Triggers
What exactly causes a migraine still isn't fully understood, however, there are some factors that are often associated with the triggering of a migraine. Listed below are some of the common triggers.
Common triggers of migraine include:
- Stress
- Hormones
- Strong scents
- Anxiety
- Lack of sleep
- Skipped meals
- Low blood sugar

- Smoke
- Weather conditions
- Food allergies
- Certain foods
- Blood pressure
- The pill
- Medication

a) Stress
Stress is a well-known cause of migraines and many sufferers report that they have more of these distressing attacks when they are under periods of stress. New research shows that migraines can occur when a stressful period comes to an end, something researchers call a "stress let-down".
A person can endure a stressful period with no symptoms of a migraine and then suffer a migraine when that stressful period comes to an end.

b) Hormones
Some women find that their migraines are more frequent at certain times of the cycle. Hormones can occur more before a period, or sometimes during or afterwards.
A hormone imbalance can often result in fluctuations in the blood sugar, and this will also cause migraines in some people. There is a chapter later on in the book about addressing hormonal imbalances.

c) Strong scents
Strong scents can be a common trigger among migraine sufferers. Other sensory stimulation such as flickering lights or flashing lights can also trigger them in some patients.

d) Anxiety
Some patients experience frequent migraines during periods of anxiety. Finding ways of effectively managing anxiety such as

meditation, yoga or CBT are all helpful methods to reduce this type of stress.

e) Insomnia

Insomnia or periods of unsettled sleep can be a contributor to migraines and some patients will experience insomnia when they have had a migraine. In order to tackle insomnia, patients need to develop a regular routine at bedtime and address any issues that might be contributing to the poor sleep pattern.

Insomnia can also be common when the hormone levels surge.

f) Skipped Meals

Skipping meals will cause the blood sugar to run too low, and low blood sugar has been associated with headaches and migraines. Three well-balanced meals that are low in sugar, salt and fat should be eaten every day and a snack containing complex carbohydrates should be eaten in-between meals.

While many experts advise not eating late at night, a light snack just before bedtime can help to keep the blood sugar steady throughout the night and into the next morning. If you often wake up with a migraine or headache then try having a snack before bed and see if this helps.

g) Low blood sugar

Some patients find that they are more prone to these types of migraines when their blood sugars are running too low. If your migraines occur when you have gone a few hours without eating, on days when you have skipped meals or when you eat a late lunch or dinner, then it is worth considering that your blood sugar level might be contributing to the migraines. Never go more than two hours without eating something. If you feel sweaty, shaky, or excessively hungry when you haven't eaten for a while, then these are sure signs of a low blood sugar. There is a chapter later on in the book with tips to balance the blood sugars.

Chapter 1) Migraines

h) Smoke
For some people smoky atmospheres can trigger an attack. If you share a home with someone that smokes, then use an ioniser to keep the air fresher and keep windows open to keep the rooms from becoming too stale.

i) Weather
Weather conditions can trigger an attack in some patients. If it's a blazing hot day and the sun is extremely bright, then this can cause some patients to experience a migraine.

j) Food allergies
Doctors often advise keeping a food diary to see if there are any patterns. If a patient regularly experiences migraines after eating certain foods than this could be the sign of an allergy or intolerance to certain foods.

k) Certain foods
Foods such as cheese, chocolate, excessively salty foods and wine are all common migraine triggers. When it comes to diet, eat as naturally as possible, prepare meals from scratch where you can, and avoid excessive amounts of preservatives.

l) Blood pressure
High blood pressure has been known to trigger migraines and patients should be checked for this if they are having regular attacks. Patients with high blood pressure will usually be given diet advice and blood pressure medication will be prescribed if changing the diet isn't enough.

m) Hormones
Migraines are more common among women and many believe that there is a hormonal link. Some women experience more of these migraines when they are taking oral contraception.

Chapter 1) Migraines

n) Medication
Some medications can trigger migraines in patients and people that regularly take pain medication are also more vulnerable to headaches/migraines. It is not uncommon for patients that consistently take medication to develop headaches.

o) Exercise
For some people exercise can trigger a migraine. This usually occurs when a person undertakes strenuous activity that they are not used to or if they exercise for longer and harder than they normally would.

Chapter 2) Medications and Treatments for Migraines

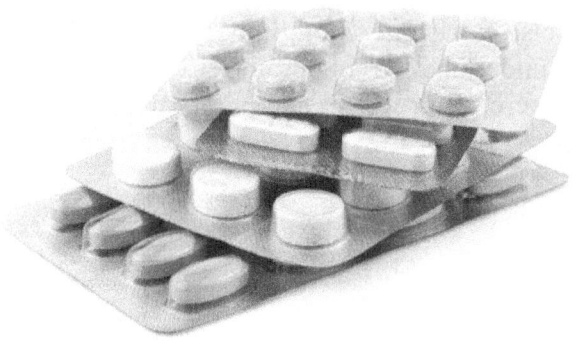

1) Medication

Depending on the severity of the pain, over-the-counter medications might be enough for a patient to manage some of their symptoms. The most commonly used over-the-counter medicines are paracetomol and Ibuprofen. These medicines should not be relied upon for on-going treatment as they can both lead to rebound headaches; these types of headaches often occur when a patient regularly takes medication to help manage everyday head pain and can make migraines worse in some patients.

If buying over-the-counter medicine, then there are several factors that need to be taken into consideration. If you are on any other type of medication then you should ask to speak to a pharmacist to make sure the medication you are buying won't interact with any other drugs you are taking.

Moreover, some types of medications can make the effects of alcohol stronger or they might make a person drowsy so a patient should avoid driving. Make sure that you check all of this before using over- the-counter preparations and if the medication does

Chapter 2) Medications and Treatments for Migraines

not prove effective as a migraine treatment, then speak to your doctor/physician.

This chapter details just some of the common medical treatments that are offered to migraine sufferers.

There are also details of some of the most common side effects, but the list is by no means exhaustive. Full details of any potential side effects will be detailed on an information leaflet that comes with the medication.

Anti-inflammatory, over-the-counter medications come in various forms such as tablets or liquid. Detailed below are some of the most common over-the-counter medications that can be used to help treat the pain caused by migraine.

1) When to take medication

Migraine medication should be taken as soon as possible as this is when it is at its most effective. Don't be tempted to try and delay taking medication for as long as possible, take it as soon as you start experiencing the symptoms of a migraine.

Medications to manage the nausea that is associated with migraines should also be taken as soon as possible before the symptoms are allowed to worsen.

2) Frequent Attacks

Once a patient has experienced a migraine it makes them much more likely to experience another one. Some sufferers can get to the point where they are either having the symptoms of a migraine attack or having a full migraine attack every day, therefore it is important that a patient works with their doctor to find the right medications to both manage a migraine and to prevent them.

3) Ibuprofen

This medication is available in several forms and all of the major drug manufacturers have their version of it. It is also available as

Chapter 2) Medications and Treatments for Migraines

a generic brand and supermarkets often sell own brand versions. It is available in 200mg and 400mg doses; some doctors suggest beginning with the lower dose, and then using a higher dose if this does not prove effective.

Moreover, there are some medications containing ibuprofen that are available especially for migraine sufferers, these often contain an ingredient called lysine as well.

Several "express" formulas and soluble formulas are also available and these are useful for quick pain relief.

Side Effects:

The most common side effects of ibuprofen is bleeding, so patients are advised not to take this type of medication long term. It can also cause digestive upsets and if a patient is on blood thinning medication then it is likely they will be advised not to take it without careful monitoring of their GP.

4) Naproxen

Naproxen will have an anti-inflammatory and pain killing effect and may be suggested for patients that don't find ibuprofen effective. Naproxen is stronger than ibuprofen, although some patients find that it takes longer to work than other anti-inflammatories. Naproxen is often prescribed by a doctor, but it is available as an over-the-counter medication in 500mg doses. Naproxen shouldn't be taken without speaking to your doctor first as it can interact with other medications.

Side Effects:

As with other anti-inflammatories, Naproxen can cause stomach problems and some patients find it causes minor side effects such as skin problems or itchiness and some patients experience a dry mouth.

5) Nurofen Migraine Pain

This medication has been made available as an over-the-counter medication for the fast treatment of migraines. The active

Chapter 2) Medications and Treatments for Migraines

ingredient is ibuprofen lysine and it has been designed to get to work quickly to alleviate a migraine.
In addition, Nurofen also have an express version of this product. The active ingredient in this medication is Sodium Ibuprofen and it is suitable for migraine sufferers.
Side Effects:
See Ibuprofen.
Supermarkets also sell their own brands of Ibuprofen and some patients will find these to be every bit as effective, however, look at the amount of active ingredients before buying.

6) Aspirin

For minor pain, an aspirin may be adequate to help relieve the pain that is associated with migraine.
Quick acting formulas are available so the medication will get to work straight away and relieve the symptoms much quicker.
Side Effects
The most common side effect of taking aspirin is the possibility that it can cause bleeding of the stomach. Patients on blood thinning medication are usually advised to be careful when taking aspirin and would be well advised to speak to their consultant/physician before taken aspirin.
Moreover, aspirin might not be suitable for long-term use.

7) Paracetomol

Paracetomol is another effective drug for migraine pain. Patients are advised to take the medication as soon as possible into an attack in order to get the most benefit from it.
As well as being available in tablet form, it can be brought as a soluble version, which some people might find acts quicker.
Paracetomol is available as a branded or generic medication. All of the supermarkets sell their own brands; these are much cheaper than other brands and are often as effective.

Chapter 2) Medications and Treatments for Migraines

Paracetomol can also be brought as Panadol, and many patients find this an effective means of pain control. Panadol extra is available in both tablet and soluble form and Panadol ultra-tablets are also used for migraines. There is also a night time formula that can be used for migraines.

Side Effects

This drug is considered safe to take for most people but some patients experience a fall in blood pressure or hypo-tension and excessive amounts of this medication have been linked with kidney and liver disease.

8) Migraleve

Migraleve is readily available from supermarkets and chemists. The pills comes in two different colours, pink and yellow, and each is designed to treat the different stages of a migraine. The pink tablets contain codeine and paracetomol, as well as a drug called buclizine to reduce nausea and the yellow tablets contain codeine and paracetomol.

Side Effects:

The most common side effects of codeine are dizziness, feelings of drowsiness and some patients can experience problems with a shortness of breath.

The following medications are just some of the possible treatment options that a doctor/physician might prescribe for the treatment of migraine

Antiemetics might also be prescribed to help address the symptoms of sickness and nausea.

9) Verapamil

As well as being prescribed for the treatment of migraine, this drug is also used as a treatment for patients with cluster headaches. The drug is known to reduce the amount of attacks in some patients and it is an effective medication for helping migraine sufferers to manage their attacks; the drug is usually taken three times a day.

Chapter 2) Medications and Treatments for Migraines

Side Effects:
Most of the side effects of this drug are minor. Side effects can include light headedness, numbness and itching; some patients report a rash while taking this drug. However, some patients say that they don't have any side effects when taking verapamil.

10) Triptans

Triptans come in many different forms and are available in over-the-counter medications. Products such as Imagran Recovery include Sumitriptan as its active ingredient and the medication is available over the counter. Imagran Recovery comes in tablet form, injections and as a nasal spray.

11) Migard

Other triptan-based medications include Migard. Migard includes Frovatriptan as its active ingredient and the medication can be used as a spray or tablets, Another product, Zomig, contains zolmitriptan as its active ingredient.

Products like Migard will be active for up to 26 hours so patients prefer this type of medication if they have a special event to get through and they don't want their day ruined by a migraine.

Migard – Side effects:
Most of the side effects of Migard are usually minor and include a dry mouth or problems with the digestion. Some patients might also experience problems such as a tight chest after taking this medication.

Contraindications:
Migard is not suitable for all patients, especially if they have an underlying condition such as a heart problem. Patients should consult with a GP/physician first before taking this type of medication.

Chapter 2) Medications and Treatments for Migraines

12) Amitriptyline

This is an anti-depressant medication but it is commonly prescribed for chronic pain such as nerve pain; however, it is also used as an effective medication for preventing migraines.
Side Effects:
Some people experience problems concentrating, a skin rash, tiredness and tingling.

13) Pizotifen

This medication is prescribed for preventing migraine. This medication is usually used to help treat migraines in young people.
Side Effects:
Some patients report weight gain while taking this medication due to the increase in appetite that Pizotifen can sometimes cause. A dry mouth and feelings of nausea can also be common when taking this medication.

14) Topiramate

Also known as Topamax, this medication is often used to treat seizures; however, it can also be prescribed for patients with migraines. Some patients don't like the bitter taste of the medication, so it is suggested that it is taken with sugar or something sweet to help overcome the taste.
Side Effects:
Like many other medications, Topiramate can cause side effects. Some of the side effects include stomach upsets and problems with digestion, a dry mouth and problems swallowing.

15) Propranolol

This medication is known for its effects on the blood vessels so it is sometimes prescribed for the treatment of migraines. Propranolol is a beta blocker and is commonly prescribed to help

people manage anxiety attacks and blood pressure problems, as well as for migraines.
Side Effects:
The most common side effects include stomach upsets, problems sleeping and over tiredness. More severe affects can include changes in the heart rate and pains in the chest.

16) Imitrex

Imitrex is sometimes suggested by specialists as an effective treatment for migraines, however, the drug is expensive and while some people find it effective, it will not prevent a migraine and should only be taken once a migraine has started.
Imitrex is used for patients that have migraines with or without aura and it is also effective for nausea. This drug can be used as a nasal spray.
This drug can have interactions with other medications and there are many contraindications for this medication, so it should not be taken without medical supervision.
Side Effects:
This drug can cause nausea, tiredness and minor headaches in some patients.

17) Blood Pressure Medication

Some patients with high blood pressure can also be prone to migraines so blood pressure medication is prescribed to help relieve the symptoms.
The type of blood pressure medication that a doctor prescribes will depend on a patient's medical history and the other types of medication that a patient might be on.
It is also likely that the patient's GP will want to monitor the patient's blood pressure to make sure that the medication is working and this will usually require regular appointments with the doctor or a practice nurse.

Chapter 2) Medications and Treatments for Migraines

2) Other Ways of Finding Pain Relief

Medical manufactures are always developing new medications. By getting involved in clinical trials, patients can benefit from the newest medications; however, patients also need to be aware that these studies are not without risk.

Finding databases of current trials is quite straight forward. Sites such as the World Health Organisation have a database of current clinical trials. Migraine sufferers – and sufferers of any other disease – only need to do a basic search and a list of trials will come up.

However, getting involved in a clinical study can involve a lot of travelling and the studies can sometimes go on for years; they'll often require frequent visits to the hospital/clinic for monitoring and tests, so clinical trials won't be suitable for everyone. Clinical trials that are underway at the time of writing include a Botox trial and a non-invasive stimulation device.

The criteria for clinical trials is very strict and they are often not available to people over a certain age group or undergoing some types of medical treatment. For instance, the trial involving a non-invasive stimulation device is not open to patients who are being treated with Botox.

The following methods of pain control only tend to be used when all other preventative and treatment methods have been used but the patient still hasn't experienced relief from their symptoms.

a) Nerve Block Injections

If other types of medications aren't working, and if the migraines are persistent, then a nerve block injection might be suggested. These injections are safe and side effects are rare, however, patients might experience some tenderness at the injection site afterwards, but using ice will help to reduce this.

For patients that don't like needles, or patients who are just unsure about the procedure and feel anxious about it, then a sedative will be offered.

Chapter 2) Medications and Treatments for Migraines

b) Botox

Botox is used for the treatment of chronic migraines; migraines are considered chronic if a patient suffers from them for more than 15 days of every month.

Botox is more commonly used in the United States to treat migraines and it is only available to patients in the UK if they have already tried medication without success. The patient will have had to been prescribed at least three different types of medications, and if these have all failed to effectively treat the migraine, then the patient may be eligible to be considered for Botox treatment.

Botox treatments aren't used as the first line of treatment and it will usually only be considered if a patient is unable to manage their symptoms any other way.

c) Occipital Nerve Stimulation

This therapy has been shown to be beneficial for the treatment of chronic migraine; however, Occipital nerve stimulation has only been shown to be effective in the short-term.

Occipital nerve stimulation is carried out in two different stages and there is a risk of complications from this type of surgery.

d) Trans cranial Magnetic Stimulation (TMS)

TMS has recently been approved for the treatment and prevention of migraines for sufferers in the UK. This form of therapy is used while the patient is experiencing an aura before a migraine attack or at the start of a migraine.

The aim of the treatment is to prevent attacks and reduce the frequency of the migraines.

TMS offers a non-invasive approach to preventing and treating migraines and placing a device on the scalp that is used to deliver trans cranial magnetic stimulation and the device can also be used alongside other medications.

e) Migraine Clinics

If a patient doesn't respond to medication, then it might be suggested that they attend a migraine clinic. A patient is also

Chapter 2) Medications and Treatments for Migraines

likely to be referred to a migraine clinic if they have one of the rarer types of migraines or if they are suffering from increasingly severe migraines.

Migraine clinics are held throughout the UK and patients can be referred privately if they wish.

Chapter 3) Treating Migraines Naturally

When it comes to healthcare, there are plenty of people that don't want to be dependent on medication and prefer a more natural approach to coping with their symptoms.
Over the years, research has shown several vitamins, minerals and herbs to be an effective way of managing migraines. Likewise, natural therapies such as acupuncture or aromatherapy might be beneficial for a patient. People who find that being stressed can cause a migraine can find aromatherapy especially useful and massage therapy is also a good option if tight muscles in the neck area trigger a migraine.
If one form of therapy or natural treatment doesn't work for you, then don't be scared to try something else and keep trying until you find something that does ease your symptoms.

In this chapter, you'll find a number of suggestions for natural treatments for migraines and for their symptoms. However, before trying any of them discuss these alternative therapies with your medical team in case any of the therapies detailed in this chapter have a contraindication with any medication that you might be taking for your migraines or for any other health condition.

1) Vitamins

a) Magnesium
Magnesium is often recommended for migraine sufferers due to the effects it can have on the vessels, although more research is needed into how effective the mineral is. When a person suffers a migraine, the vessels in the brain constrict, magnesium relaxes

these vessels and many patients find that this essential mineral can help their symptoms.

Magnesium can be taken as a supplement and it is best taken alongside calcium and boron, so look for a supplement that contains all three of these minerals. However, patients should also be aware that taking extra magnesium can cause stomach upsets in some people when it is taken in large doses.

This mineral is also useful if you have problems sleeping at night as magnesium will help you to relax, and lack of sleep can contribute to a migraine. For night time use, take a supplement an hour or so before bed, or try one of the magnesium sprays last thing at night.

Adding magnesium to the diet

To include extra magnesium in the diet without supplementing, eat lots of green leafy vegetables, nuts and seeds.

b) B2

Research has shown that B2 or riboflavin could be an effective way of treating migraines, although more research is needed. Riboflavin has also been shown to be effective at lessening the number of cluster headache attacks in some patients when given in supplements of 400mg a day, however, excessive amounts of vitamins should not be taken without speaking to a medical professional first.

To supplement the diet with B2, take it as part of a B complex to make sure that you get healthy levels of all of the B vitamins. To get B vitamins in your diet include plenty of cereals, breads, bananas and whole grains.

Contraindications:

Many drugs, including anti-depressants, can interact with B2 supplements so take medical advice if you are on any kind of medication or if you have an underlying health condition.

c) B6, B12 and Folic Acid

Studies have shown that when these vitamins are taken in combination patients experience less severe migraines and it can reduce the frequency of attacks.

This is because these supplements can reduce the homocysteine levels in the body. Homocysteine is an amino acid that is produced when the body breaks down proteins in the body, however, high levels of homocysteine can cause inflammation.

d) B12 Injections

Some migraine patients respond well to B12 injections. Patients deficient in the vitamin find that when they have B12 injections, then their migraines become much less frequent.

If your doctor suspects a B12 deficiency then they will arrange tests and if a B12 injection is deemed necessary then they will usually be given every few months, or more often depending on the severity of the deficiency.

e) Serra Enzyme

This is an enzyme that has an anti-inflammatory action and can help to reduce pain. As well as being used for head pain, this supplement is also useful for other inflammatory conditions such as sports injuries, overuse injuries such as Carpal Tunnel Syndrome and arthritis.

The product can be brought as Serrapeptase; it comes in various strengths and it is readily available to buy online.

Contraindications:

This supplement should not be taken by patients who are using blood thinning medication.

Side Effects:

Some patients can have an allergic reaction to the product. There are also reports of lung inflammation and liver problems in some patients, but these are rare.

Chapter 3) Treating Migraines Naturally

f) Co enzyme Q10

Co enzyme Q10 has often been used to promote heart health and it is also believed to help diabetics to help better control their blood sugar levels. However, it has also shown promise as a treatment for migraines and side effects are usually rare.

Side Effects:

The most common side effects are stomach upsets and digestive problems.

Contraindications:

Co enzyme Q10 can lower blood pressure so it shouldn't be taken by patients with low blood pressure or patients on blood pressure medication. It should also not be taken by patients on cancer drugs or patients on blood thinning medication.

It is also advisable that pregnant women don't take Co Enzyme Q10 as there is a lack of research into any possible harm it could cause.

2) Herbs

a) Feverfew

This herb has long been suggested as a treatment for migraine sufferers; however more studies are needed into just how effective feverfew is. This is a herb that grows relatively easily so some patients like to cultivate their own, however, for most people it is a better idea to buy standardised supplements and to follow the directions for the exact amount to take each day.

If you do grow your own feverfew then the herb can be incorporated in the diet easily by adding it to salads and sandwiches.

Side Effects:

Feverfew is generally considered safe, but some people can experience a swelling in the lips and mouth. Other symptoms such as digestive difficulties have also been reported. In addition, it is not a good idea to take feverfew long term has it can cause more severe side effects such as insomnia and stiff joints.

Chapter 3) Treating Migraines Naturally

Pregnant women should not take feverfew and some people are allergic to the shrub.

h) Butterbur
Butterbur is a shrub that grows in Europe; it can also be found in Asia and North America. It has shown potential for the treatment of many health maladies including headaches and migraine and studies have shown that butterbur can indeed be effective at helping to manage migraines.
However, there is also some evidence that the shrub could cause damage to the liver; this is because of a substance in butterbur called pyrrolizidine alkaloids. For this reason only products that are labelled as free from this ingredient should be purchased.

c) Willow Bark
Willow bark has an ingredient called Salicin. When this ingredient is broken down in the body, it is turned into salicylic acid, which is often used to help relieve pain.

d) Raspberry Leaf
Raspberry leaf is often taken by pregnant women to help ease nausea during pregnancy but it can be useful for other types of nausea as well. If the migraines are triggered by hormones, then raspberry leaf is a good option as it is believed to help balance the hormones.
Raspberry leaf can be brought as a dried herb, a tea or as capsules.
Contraindications:
Although pregnant women often drink raspberry tea to help ease labour pains there are some contraindications and these should be discussed with your GP/Practitioner before supplementing the diet with it.

e) Ginger
Ginger is a traditional remedy to stop nausea, but it can also be used to treat headaches, too. It can be used as a tea, in capsule

form, or some people prefer to eat crystallised ginger or ginger biscuits.

Side Effects:

Ginger isn't usually known to cause side effects; however, consuming excessive amounts of ginger can cause stomach upsets and heartburn.

Contraindications:

Patients on diabetes or blood thinning medication should take advice before supplementing with ginger. Patients using blood medication or patients with high blood pressure should speak to a doctor/practitioner before adding ginger to their diet.

3) Natural Therapies

As well as supplements, there are many different forms of complimentary therapy that migraine patients find useful. The effectiveness of these therapies will vary for everyone, but many say that using complimentary therapy has been extremely beneficial in helping to treat and manage their migraines.

a) Acupuncture

Many patients find that acupuncture can help to reduce the frequency and intensity of migraines. Although the thought of having needles applied to the skin won't appeal to some people it is usually a painless process and if a patient feels any pain during a session they should tell the practitioner and they will move the needle to a different position.

When it comes to treating head pain, the needles are usually placed on the ear, head or body, but the positioning will vary depending on the patient's symptoms.

Sessions usually last an hour and there might be some minor side effects such as light headedness or some slight bruising from the needle after a treatment session. Patients are advised to have a light snack before having acupuncture.

It will often take several sessions before a patient will start to see an improvement in their symptoms. It may be necessary to attend up to ten treatments before noticing a reduction in migraines.

b) Physiotherapy

Physiotherapy or physical therapy is useful for treating migraines in some patients. If neck tension is one of your common migraine triggers, then regular sessions with a therapist will often be very beneficial.

After taking down some notes on your medical history, the therapist will examine you. They will usually suggest using some massage techniques to reduce any tension that has gathered in the neck area and they will also look at other factors that can contribute to migraine such as shoulder tension.

A therapist might also do some manipulation techniques to help free up the neck and the shoulder area. Some patients might find that they feel light headed after massage and manipulation – this is just where the tension has been released and the head feels lighter because of it.

Patients might also notice some discomfort after a session of massage; this shouldn't be too severe and will settle down after a couple of days.

As well as physio or physical therapy, migraine sufferers might also find that osteopathy or a session with a chiropractor would be useful to help free up joints and muscles and to reduce tension, reducing pain throughout the head and the body and freeing up the body so that it is easier to move.

c) Trigger Point Therapy

Sometimes pain in the head can come from somewhere else in the body. For instance, if you suffer from migraines or head pain, then it might be triggered by a point in your neck or shoulder.

A trigger point can be best described as tight muscle tissue; this tight muscle tissue can refer the pain to somewhere else in the body. This type of referred pain can cause pain all over the body. What starts out as a pain in the back, could soon cause pain in the neck or shoulder area, in turn, this could then trigger pain in the head.

Chapter 3) Treating Migraines Naturally

A trigger point therapist will work with a patient to find these tight areas of muscle or knots. This can sometimes cause some discomfort during a session and the patient might also feel some pain afterwards. However, some patients won't experience any pain at all; it just depends on the individual.

If a patient does experience some pain following a treatment session then ice can be used to help ease the discomfort.

For patients who notice that they have pain somewhere else in the body, it is a good idea to find out if the pain is being referred and contributing to a migraine or head pain.

d) The Dorn Method and Migraines

Many people won't be familiar with this form of natural therapy as it is not as well-known as some of the others. Here, Paul Knowles, an advanced Dorn Method Practitioner explains more about the therapy and how it can help patients with migraines:

"The Dorn Method has been named after its founder Dieter Dorn. It is a Complementary Therapy that has been developed over the last 40 years with its origins in Germany.

The Dorn Method was originally developed to help relieve Back & Joint pain, but has been found useful in helping many other ailments both mental & physical.

This is due to the way it works on the Meridians & Nervous System by re-aligning the vertebrae of the Spine.

I have personally found The Dorn Method to be very successful in relieving Migraines in my clients for many years now.

I have found that most of my clients who have reported suffering with Migraines to have misaligned Cervical vertebrae such as C1 & C2.

These vertebrae place pressure upon the nerves causing them to become inflamed.

This inflammation causes tension to build up at the base of the skull resulting in Headaches & Migraines.

By gently releasing these misaligned vertebrae and placing them back into their natural positions using the techniques of The Dorn Method, pressure is taken off the nerves and tension is released allowing the inflammation to subside which caused the Migraine

Chapter 3) Treating Migraines Naturally

to become present causing the client severe pain.

All Dorn Method corrections happen in a dynamic way, that is, with the client helping the Therapy by actively participating with the Practitioner.

Dorn is very safe and free from unpleasant side effects. No medication is required.

Each Dorn Method session takes 1 hour.

Regarding how long before a client notices a difference, I have known people that have felt better after just a 10 minutes treatment to people that have noticed a difference a couple of days after Dorn sessions."

e) Osteopathy

Tim Allardyce, MCSP SRP, is an Osteopath at Croydon Physio. He explains what to expect when you visit an osteopath for treatment for the first time and how an osteopath can help in the treatment of headaches and the related symptoms.

"An osteopath will look at your body in a holistic way, to work out the cause of your pain. Osteopaths believe that everything in the body is there for a reason, and is underpinned by three philosophies: 1) Structure governs function (meaning that the structure of the body is there for a purpose, for a function). 2) The rule of the artery is supreme – if we normalise blood flow in the body, we will stimulate healing as blood delivers oxygen and metabolites necessary for cell repair. 3) The body produces its own medicines, and is capable of self-healing if given the right conditions."

"During your first treatment we will take a case history. This involves asking you questions about how your injury/pain occurred, when it occurred, which things make it worse, and which things make it better. We will also ask you about sports, work and hobbies that you do that might affect your condition. We will also ask about your previous medical history, such as serious illnesses, or previous similar problems. After this, we will do a physical examination. This includes looking at your muscles and bone structure, posture, and checking your range of movement. We might ask you to bend, side-bend, or rotate to

Chapter 3) Treating Migraines Naturally

check how mobile your joints are. We will also palpate your muscles to determine how tight they are."

"Once the examination is complete, we will discuss with you what the diagnosis is, and how the condition is most effectively treated. Assuming that no further tests or examinations are required, treatment will then commence, and usually involves manual hands-on therapy."

Tim also explains how osteopathy is used to treat headaches. "The first question that needs to be asked by your osteopath is: "what is causing the headaches". It could be that a certain food allergy, stress or psychological illness, hormones, posture, or muscle tension is the causative factor. If your osteopath feels that the neck, posture, or muscle tension is the cause, they will treat the relevant area to relive your headaches. A significant number of headaches can be attributed to the neck. When neck muscles get tight, it can restrict blood flow to the head, and also pinch on nerves going to the head causing the pain of headaches. There is a particularly naughty group of muscles that sit just below the back of the skull called the suboccipital muscles. This group of four small muscles can get very tight, causing referred pain into the back of the head and then over to the eyes and frontal part of the head."

"We are also seeing an increased prevalence of office workers suffering headaches, especially those who spend long hours with their neck bent forwards. Computer monitors are a big problem too, when they are too low it places the neck in a poor postural position, placing strain on the neck muscles and ligaments. Laptop use is the other big cause, encouraging people to bend their neck forwards. Another common cause is stress, as the muscles in the neck tighten when we are tense, especially when hunching our shoulders."

So how do we treat your headaches?

"We have many techniques in our tool box to use to relieve your headaches. The most common is massage to release muscle tension in the head and neck. The second is joint mobilisation. When the neck is stiff, you are more likely to suffer headaches, so improving range of mobility to your neck using manual

Chapter 3) Treating Migraines Naturally

techniques can reduce your headaches. Sometimes we use traction, to stretch the neck, and relieve pressure on the joints, discs, and muscles. We will also look at ways of improving your posture. Typically people with bad posture will more likely suffer headaches as the neck is put into a mechanically poor position. This is known as forward head posture, and puts the neck under enormous strain. By correcting posture with soft tissue techniques and exercises, we can relieve the strain on your head. Other tools sometimes used include acupuncture, and ultrasound."

But that is not all we will do:

"Being holistic practitioners, we will look to discuss ways to improve your lifestyle. So we might need you to change your workstation set up, or cut out certain foods in your diet, or do exercises to strengthen your neck, or give you strategies to reduce stress. All of these combined with treatment to your neck can make a super powerful natural headache cure. I cure about 90% of headaches using these techniques, so you can see that it's very successful as a form of treatment, and also very safe without the need for medication."

6 top tips to fix headaches:
- Use a laptop stand – for less than £30 you can raise your laptop and it puts less strain through the neck.
- Raise your monitor by 4 inches – it will help keep you upright, and stop your neck bending forwards so much.
- Use a document holder to stop repetitive forward neck bending and extending. Keeping your documents at eye level will reduce the constant bending and extending.
- Hold your iPad and iPhone up high when using them for long periods.
- Reduce stress – suboccipital muscles are affected by stress, so reducing stress can reduce the tension in these muscles. Learn to relax your shoulders to reduce the tension in the neck muscles.
- See an osteopath or physiotherapist, many have experience treating headaches.

Chapter 3) Treating Migraines Naturally

f) Aromatherapy

Using essential oils can be an effective way to reduce migraines, however, migraine sufferers shouldn't use oils that are too strongly scented or they can actually make headaches worse. Essential oils can be added to water, massaged into the skin, provided they are mixed with base oil, or dropped onto the pillow. It is suggested that pregnant women or breastfeeding women don't use them without speaking to a doctor first and patients with epilepsy should also be careful when it comes to using some of the oils.

As there can be some contraindications, it is a good idea to speak to your doctor/physician if you have any other health problems or if you are taking medication.

The use of essential oils can be extremely beneficial in reducing stress and tension. If stress is a major contributor to your migraines then oils such as lavender and camomile can be useful as they are well known for their calming effects.

Try using the oils last thing at night to prevent insomnia or at stressful times to try and counter tension.

Essential oils can also be useful for managing symptoms such as nausea. Peppermint is known to reduce nausea and digestive upsets; ginger can also help reduce feeling of sickness.

g) Chiropractor

A chiropractor can be helpful in helping to relieve migraines, or at least reduce the number of attacks. If a patient is prone to migraines because of muscle tension in the neck area, then this form of treatment may well be very beneficial. Other hands of manipulation therapies such as osteopathy might also be useful for patients that carry excess tension in the neck area and if poor posture contributes to the problem, then other natural therapies like the Alexander Technique may be useful.

h) Biofeedback

Biofeedback helps a person to gain a greater understanding and awareness of the various physiological functions of the body. This

Chapter 3) Treating Migraines Naturally

can help patients to address issues such as muscle tension; biofeedback is a technique often used by physiotherapists. However, various devices are available such as the iRelax system or the EmWave 2 and these can be used at home, but should not be used without first speaking to a doctor

Regular use of a biofeedback device can help a patient to monitor and manage their stress levels throughout the day and while the initial cost is more expensive, it is a useful device for people that need regular therapy to cope with stress or muscle tension.

i)Massage therapy
Massage is an excellent remedy for a migraine. Facial massage is ideal and can be easily performed daily. Detailed below are some massage techniques for dealing with migraines:

Go underneath on the back of the neck and feel a hollow, which is centered on the back between the ears. Put pressure on this hollow underneath the skull base.

Place your thumbs on either side of the bridge of your nose right at the base, where it joins the forehead. Squeeze the bridge by pushing the thumbs towards each other. Apply firm pressure, but no pain. Hold for ten seconds and repeat about three to five times. Keep the thumbs in same place on the nose bridge, but rotate so that your thumb pads face towards the forehead. Press upward with thumbs and hold for ten seconds. Repeat this a few times.

Now, finish with some head and neck stretches. Slowly tilt your head on one side, going all the way and lowering your ear to the shoulder. Relax for ten seconds. Then, slowly raise your head and repeat on the other side. Next, drop your chin down into your chest. Relax for ten seconds. Allow your head to slowly fall towards your back this time and repeat.

Aromatherapy is a powerful treatment and can be combined with massage. There are quite a few essential oils to utilize with a migraine. First, there is lavender essential oil. Of all the essential oils, lavender can be used neat (no need to dilute with a base oil). Just dab some on your temples and try a warm bath with added drops for a restful night's sleep. Other essential oils for migraines are coriander, peppermint, rosemary, marjoram, chamomile, clary

Chapter 3) Treating Migraines Naturally

sage, angelica, rose Otto and Melissa (lemon balm oil). Use those with a base oil, such as olive oil and massage into your temples, forehead and into your hairline.

Blends can be created with olive oil, using lavender, peppermint, chamomile, etc. Also massage the oil blends over your solar plexus (upper abdomen), in addition to your head and temples.

Buy an unperfumed base cream and add several drops of lavender to the cream. Apply to temples and back of neck as needed.

J) Crystal Healing

Crystal Healing isn't for everyone, and many would argue that they only act as a placebo, however, some people do swear by them, and the placebo effect can be a powerful one.

Here, a crystal healing specialist explains how she uses crystals to help treat the symptoms of a migraine.

"I have often used crystals and have found that you really can feel better with them. Just carrying a rose quartz stone often makes my day! Crystals can also help with physical ailments, such as migraines. Try this technique. You will need one smoky quartz, one carnelian, two serpentines, and one amethyst.

Place the quartz on the floor just below where your feet should be, when you lie down.

Lie down and get comfortable.

Place a carnelian on your lower abdomen.

Place one serpentine at center of your chest, over your heart and place the other one over your throat.

Place the amethyst right above your head.

Continue to lie comfortable and still. Relax like this for at least five to six minutes. Then, remove the stones and repeat, whenever needed.

You can also carry the stones with you, when at work, home, etc. Jewelry made from genuine crystals are ideal for this".

Chapter 4) Food Triggers, Diet and Nutrition

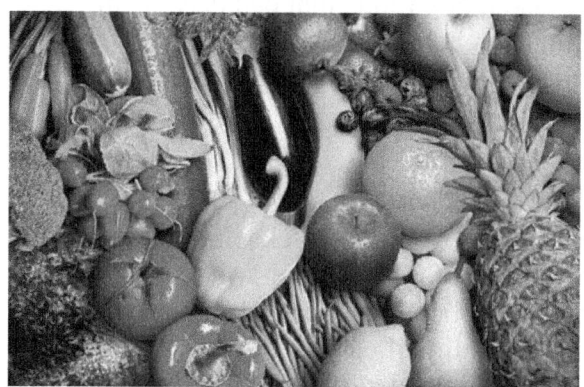

Food triggers are extremely common in migraine sufferers and many sufferers find that when they change their diet and leave out certain foods or additives, that they experience less migraines, however, the food triggers will be different for everyone. For instance, some people find that having caffeine can help to prevent head pain, while others find that their migraines/headaches worsen when they consume too much caffeine.

Some experts suggest carrying out an elimination diet to help pinpoint the foods that are triggering the attacks and details of how to do this are detailed later on in this chapter, but it is a good idea to speak to a medical expert before doing this to ensure that you don't exclude vital nutrients from the diet.

Another good idea is to keep a diary to track migraine attacks, along with any medication that might be being used, the foods that you eat and the events that are going on as this will make it easier to spot patterns and to find what is causing and triggering your attacks.

Nutrition can play a vital role in helping to prevent migraines as it can help to prevent low blood sugars, hormone imbalances, and provide vital nutrients to the body, so detailed below are some tips on how to use foods to treat migraines.

Chapter 4) Food Triggers, Diet and Nutrition

1) Healing Migraines with Nutrition

Recent studies have shown that there is a shocking link between migraines and food. There are many foods that can *cause* migraines and there are also many foods that can *cure* them. Below is a brief guide that can help you to determine what is triggering your migraines and which foods you can consume to cure yourself of them.

2) The Food and Migraine Link

A group of researchers at the Hospital for Sick Children located in London conducted a study on 88 individuals who suffered from extreme migraines. The researchers put each individual on an elimination diet to try to determine if certain foods trigger their migraines. After they had eliminated a list of foods that were thought to trigger these headaches, 78 of the individuals recovered completely from their migraines and 4 greatly improved.

After the researchers introduced the eliminated foods all but 8 of the individuals suffered from a migraine recurrence. Since then, it has been determined that food choices can greatly influence the severity and recurrence of migraines.

3) Determine what is causing your Migraines

Before you can properly treat your migraines, you must first know what causes them. There is a long list of foods that can trigger headaches, and you must eliminate them from your diet before you can add in the foods that can cure them. Take a look below at the various types of migraine triggers and determine which one best fits your symptoms.

4) Digestive Tract Imbalances

Some migraines are caused by an imbalance in the digestive tract, which is caused by a food allergy. Below is a list of symptoms of a digestive tract imbalance and how you can determine if it is the cause of your migraines.

Chapter 4) Food Triggers, Diet and Nutrition

- **Symptoms:** achy muscles or joints, abdominal bloating, irritable bowel syndrome, brain fogginess, excessive fatigue, sinus congestion and postnasal drip.
- **The Test:** An elimination diet is the best way to begin to determine if you have a digestive tract imbalance. Yeast, dairy, eggs and gluten are common triggers and should be eliminated from your diet. After totally eliminating this list of foods from your diet for a period of 2 weeks, assess your migraines and see if they have gotten better. If they have, slowly add the eliminated foods back into your diet, one by one.

For example, add eggs back into your diet, and then reassess your migraine levels after one week. If you develop even the slightest headache, eliminate the eggs again. The second week, add dairy back into your diet and assess your tolerance. Continue doing this until you determine if any of the above listed foods trigger any headaches or migraines. If they do, you should eliminate them totally from your diet.

5) Chemical Triggers

Diets that are high in processed foods are often to blame for migraines. These foods contain many artificial preservatives in order to extend their shelf life and are often high in sodium, which can raise blood pressure levels. Increased blood pressure can trigger headaches, which can develop into migraines.

A good rule of thumb is to steer clear of any processed foods or artificially sweetened beverages. Deli meat, wine and dried fruit are also high in chemicals that can trigger migraines.

6) A Magnesium Deficiency

Magnesium is a nutrient that many individuals are deficient in. It is readily available in many fresh vegetables, but with today's hectic lifestyles, we often do not consume the recommended amounts of fresh produce that can provide us with ample amounts of magnesium.

- **Symptoms:** Muscle tightness and cramps are the main symptom of a magnesium deficiency. Other symptoms include heart palpitations, irritability, and sensitivity to loud noises, anxiety and insomnia.
- **The Test:** There are really no self-tests to perform to determine if you have a magnesium deficiency. Your doctor can perform tests to determine your red blood cell magnesium levels. However, if you are experiencing any of the above symptoms, chances are you are magnesium deficient.

Try to consume foods high in magnesium (such as bananas, kidney beans and brown rice) or take a good quality magnesium supplement.

7) Common Trigger Foods
Some foods are known to trigger migraines more than others. You should avoid these foods at all costs. They are:
- any foods that contain MSG or nitrates
- nuts and nut butters
- sourdough bread
- lima beans and snow peas
- any type of chocolate
- any type of alcohol
- citrus fruits
- excessive amounts of caffeine
- fermented or pickled foods
- sour cream
- ripened cheeses

8) Healing Foods
Now that you know which foods you may need to eliminate let's take a look at which nutrients that are found in foods that can help heal you.

Chapter 4) Food Triggers, Diet and Nutrition

Vitamin B2: Researchers have determined that vitamin B2 can reduce the recurrence of migraines by up to 50%. Adding foods such as asparagus, quinoa and crimini mushrooms to your diet can help prevent migraines from occurring.

Magnesium: As we discussed earlier, a magnesium deficiency is one of the main triggers of migraines. Consume foods such as sunflower seeds, bananas, sweet potatoes, Swiss chard and spinach to increase your levels of this migraine fighting nutrient.

Co-enzyme Q 10: This is important for blood vessel health and it also supports your mitochondria with its high antioxidant levels. Broccoli, cauliflower, eggs, and tuna are all high in co-enzyme Q 10. Aim for 3 servings of these foods per day.

Omega-3 fatty acids: Omega-3 fatty acids can help to lower the body's production of prostaglandins, which are hormone-like chemicals known to trigger migraines. Trout, sardines, herring and salmon all contain these fatty acids. Aim for 3 to 4 servings per week.

Quercetin: This is a compound which has strong anti-inflammatory properties. Consuming 20 tart cherries or drinking 6 ounces of pure cherry juice per day can greatly reduce the occurrence and severity of migraines.

Your food choices can go a long way in helping you cure yourself of debilitating migraines. Always be sure to drink plenty of water every day, steer clear of any processed foods and eat plenty of the healing foods listed above.

Keeping a migraine journal is an effective tool to help you determine which of these foods are helping you. Every time you experience a severe headache or migraine, write down the time that it occurs and all of the foods you ate that day and the day before. This can help you to make better food choices and see if you are lacking in any of the above healing foods. After you have eliminated all the trigger foods listed above and added in all of the healing ones, you should find yourself migraine- free.

Chapter 4) Food Triggers, Diet and Nutrition

Other foods that might be useful to migraine sufferers include: Spinach, barley, green leafy vegetables, ginger, turmeric, peppermint tea and especially garlic are all purported to be beneficial for migraine sufferers.

Many of these foods listed above contain magnesium, and several studies have shown migraine sufferers to be low in this mineral, while ginger and peppermint teas are good for nausea and digestion, which is sometimes affected during a migraine. Migraine sufferers should take care with spices such as turmeric, as spicy foods can be a trigger in some patients.

Chapter 5) The Hormone Link

1) Menstrual Migraines

More women than men suffer from migraines and this is perhaps because of the hormonal link. The hormonal surges that occur in a female's body before and during menstruation can trigger a migraine in some women.

Menstrual migraines will often start a few days before a period and sometimes a patient might experience a menstrual migraine during the first few days of their period.

Migraines can also be a problem during the menopause, as the body has to manage sudden swings in hormones that can trigger a migraine.

If it is suspected that the migraines are hormone related then the patient should seek medical advice. Tests can be carried out to see if the estrogen or cortisol levels are elevated; the pill might be prescribed for some cases of hormone imbalance.

Medical treatments for these types of migraines will usually involve triptan-based medication or an anti-inflammatory might be prescribed if the symptoms are less severe.

This chapter looks at some of the causes of hormone imbalance and suggests ways of countering it.

However, hormone imbalances can be extremely detrimental to health, and it is best not to try and manage it entirely by yourself. If you suspect the reason behind your migraines is hormonal, then seek medical advice.

This chapter details both the Western approach and the Eastern approach to treating hormone imbalance and the measures women can take to re-establish the balance such as reducing stress and managing their blood sugars.

2) Causes of Hormone Imbalance

Menstrual migraines are often associated with hormone imbalance and there are several factors that can contribute to this. They include:
- Stress
- Blood sugar problems
- Excess caffeine
- Chemicals
- Diet
- Excess weight

Stress will increase the cortisol levels and this in turn will cause an increase in the estrogen levels. Even just a slight imbalance in the hormone levels is enough to cause symptoms such as tiredness, poor blood sugar control, irritability and mood swings.

a) Blood Sugars

A blood sugar level imbalance will also contribute to a hormone imbalance. When the glucose level runs too low, the body will produce cortisol to boost the blood sugar levels, and an increase in cortisol will increase the estrogen levels.

b) Caffeine

Caffeine is another substance that will increase the cortisol levels, leading to an increase in the estrogen levels.

c) Chemicals

The chemicals contained within some deodorants and in the food packaging of some ready prepared meals is thought to increase estrogen levels. Chemicals included in some cosmetic products are also believed to increase estrogen.

When possible, eat freshly prepared meals rather than packaged meals that come in plastic trays and when buying cosmetic products look for items that are free from parabens and aluminium.

d) Diet
A diet high in sugar and fast release carbohydrates will all increase the estrogen levels.

e) Weight
Women who carry excess weight are more prone to have higher estrogen levels, which will contribute to PMS and leave a woman more vulnerable to migraines.

3) Readdressing the Balance
Re-establishing hormone balance depends on addressing the factors that have contributed to it. Often, this will mean learning to manage stress more effectively, eating a balanced diet that is low in sugar and refined carbohydrates and cutting out stimulants that can increase estrogen levels.

Eating a diet high in phytoestrogens is also believed to help some women with hormone imbalance. Foods such as pulses, linseeds, vegetables such as broccoli, sprouts, cauliflower and cabbages, grains and soya products can help to achieve a better balance; detailed guidelines on eating for hormone balance on detailed later on in this chapter.

4) Herbs and Vitamins for Hormone Imbalance
There are several herbs that can be highly beneficial to women with a hormone imbalance, however, care should be taken with these as they do have an influence on the hormonal system and some of the herbs can possibly increase estrogen levels. Follow a doctor's advice before supplementing the diet with any of the herbs or vitamins listed below.

a) Evening Primrose Oil
Evening primrose oil helps to reduce inflammation and can have a positive influence on the hormone levels. Taking evening primrose oil can help to reduce pain and will also have a positive

effect on the health of the skin. The supplement is also known to reduce blood clotting.

Recommended doses for evening primrose oil vary from brand to brand. So follow the directions on the label when taking this kind of supplement.

Contraindications:

Evening primrose oil should not be taken by people on blood thinning drugs.

b) Wild Yam

This herbal supplement can be useful for women that have elevated estrogen levels. Taking wild yam in the second part of the cycle can help to balance out excessive levels of estrogen in the body and can help to ease the symptoms of PMS.

Contraindications:

Women and men with a history of hormonal influenced cancers should not supplement with Wild Yam. Patients with liver problems are also advised to take advice, and patients with any other underlying health condition or on medication, should get medical advice first.

c) Agnus Castus

Agnus Castus or Chase Tree is a herbal remedy that is often suggested for the treatment of Pre Menstrual Tension. The herb has been shown to have a balancing effect on the hormone levels, thus reducing the symptoms of hormonal imbalance, which can include the occurrence of migraines.

Some women take it all month round; however, it is also effective when taken for the first two weeks of the cycle.

The benefits from taking this herbal supplement aren't usually seen for the first three months, but some women might experience an improvement in the symptoms sooner than that.

Contraindications:

Pregnant women should not take this herbal supplement without discussing it with their GP/Physician. Agnus Castus or Chase Tree should not be taken by women with a history of hormone related cancers as it is believed that the herb has estrogenic effects and can also influence progesterone levels.

d) Dong Quai
Dong Quai is often used as a tonic and a blood purifier. However, it is also thought to have an influence on hormonal balance and is often taken by women who suffer with pre-menstrual tension; it is also taken by women who are going through the menopause as it has been shown to help reduce hot flushes.
Dong Quai shouldn't be taken by women who have had breast cancer or any other hormonal influenced cancer as Donq Quai is known to have an estrogenic effect.
Patients on blood thinning drugs, medications for cancer treatment, and pregnant women should not take this herb.

5) Stress
As detailed in the first section of this chapter, stress can be a major factor in hormone imbalance, and the imbalance can cause migraines to become more frequent.
Many people don't realise that they are under stress, always being on the go and always having something to think about becomes normal and women especially don't always notice the amount of pressure that they are under.
Often, a woman won't realise that she is under stress until the symptoms become severe. For instance, a woman might start to feel burned out, or like they just can't cope with the various challenges that are asked of them every day. The only way around this is to try and strike an even balance between work and leisure time and try and re-organise the schedule so there is some time out every day.
Learning some relaxation tips is also extremely beneficial; it is best to use these techniques every day, not just during times of extreme stress. Regular relaxation, or even just taking some time out for yourself every day, will help to combat stress and help a person to feel much more able to cope with the day ahead.

Chapter 5) The Hormone Link

Relaxation doesn't need to take the form of meditation or yoga; it could just be listening to music, or enjoying a night out. Just find something that helps to manage stress effectively and that allows you to take some time out to unwind from the day's challenges. There is a chapter detailing relaxation methods and a chapter on relaxation exercises later on in the book.

6) Diet

Diet plays a major role in helping to rebalance the hormone levels. An over reliance on high sugar foods and caffeinated drinks will cause swings in the blood sugar levels that will ultimately lead to a hormonal imbalance.

However, by making a few adjustments to the diet, and by eating foods that can reduce and balance the hormones naturally, it is possible to help restore balance to the body by eating regularly and not depending on foods that contain a lot of sugar to get through the day.

Follow the steps below to help balance the female hormones and even out the blood sugars.

How to eat right to Balance Female Hormones

Other than genetics, hormonal imbalance is cause by a poor diet, often that eaten by most of the Western world. There is no particular diet for this, but there are some general rules;

- Always eat 3 meals per day. Do not skip any
- Avoid refined carbohydrates (sugar, white bread, white rice, white pasta etc.).
- Wholegrain cereals contain high levels of phytoestrogen
- Be sure to eat a minimum of 5 fruits and veg per day. Particularly green leaves and fruits high in antioxidants such as berries
- Don't try to cut fat out. Most fats are essential and very healthy, and cholesterol is a key component in transporting hormones around the body. Good fats include oily fish, nuts, yoghurt and eggs

Chapter 5) The Hormone Link

- Replace some of your carbohydrates with protein, but preferably not meat, only in moderation
- Keep caffeine consumption to a minimum, despite coffee being high in phytoestrogen... 1-2 teaspoons a day max. Caffeine can interfere with hormone regulation
- High magnesium foods such as green leafy veg will contribute to a better sleep, and so better hormone regulation
- Eat plenty of foods with lots of phytoestrogens, these include: -
    - Legumes (Inc. soybeans)
    - Brown rice
    - Seeds
    - Apples
    - Carrots
    - Oats
    - Wheat germ
- Mix coconut oil into dishes, it contains very good fats
- It may be surprising to hear, but drink beer... in moderation of course, but beer is high in phytoestrogen

7) The Eastern Approach to Hormonal Imbalance
The previous section detailed the Western approach to hormone imbalance; Chinese medicine has different theories behind how to effectively manage and achieve hormonal imbalance.
Chinese Medicine takes a completely different approach to treating hormonal imbalances, as will be described later on in this chapter; however, in order to understand Chinese medicine and how it works, this section begins with a brief explanation.

8) Understanding Chinese Medicine
The basic principle of Chinese Medical treatment is that a living human body contains vital energy (Qi) which circulates inside via discreet pathways. When these flows of energy are blocked or unbalanced, pain and illness arise. This vital energy is partly inherited from parents but must also be acquired from food and oxygen. The acquired Qi can be viewed as the essential nutrients carried by the bloodstream across the body. Given their

Chapter 5) The Hormone Link

interlinked roles, blood and Qi should be viewed collectively and in Chinese Medicine the latter is known as 'the shadow' of the former. Therefore a concept of 'lifeblood' can be helpful in understanding the Chinese Medical view that a constant circulation of energy is crucial to sustaining good health.
Tamzin Freeman, an acupuncture graduate of the College of Integrated Chinese Medicine, explains:
The Western paradigm talks about hormones - but Chinese medicine talks about Yin and Yang. With migraine the problem is generally that the Yin is deficient and the Yang rises to the head.

During the female cycle the energetics of the body change - the first half of the cycle is the Yin phase, the second half the Yang phase. The second half is when the problems generally happen, because there is too much energy that isn't being smoothly moved around, nor rooted (by the Yin). This can lead to feeling wound-up, angry and unbalanced - the energy rises to the head and causes throbbing headaches, including migraine. There may also be visual disturbance - since in Chinese medicine the eye and vision is also related to the Liver. The Liver is responsible for the smooth flow of energy around the body - and obviously this isn't happening.

It is possible to get a headache at the end of the bleed, although this is less likely to be a migraine. This is much more a deficiency headache - where the blood loss means blood deficiency which can also lead to Yin deficiency. This leads to an empty headache - this is more likely to be at the end of the day, and to go with fatigue.

Regular acupuncture aims to restore balance between Yin and Yang, and the energetics between all the organs. The most important organs to treat with gynaecological problems, and female health problems, are the Liver, the Kidneys and the Heart. However, when Chinese medicine speaks about the energetics of these organs, it doesn't mean that there is Liver, Kidney or Heart

Chapter 5) The Hormone Link

disease - the Chinese are only referring to the energy of these organs.

Here, the staff from the AcuMedic Clinic give a brief insight into Migraines and Chinese Medicine and some of the common triggers.

Common triggers of migraine include stress, anxiety, overwork, insomnia, certain foods or medications and environment - including sunlight, damp weather or cold temperature. The main symptoms of migraine are pain in one side of the head, nausea, vomiting and sensitivity to light.

Chinese Medicine distinguishes between two basic causes of migraines: external and internal. To be more precise, a Chinese Medical doctor would not focus exclusively on treating the patient's migraine, but on pinpointing the imbalance (technically known as 'the syndrome') where the cause of the migraine and other seemingly unrelated symptoms take root. Identifying the syndrome and restoring the balance will improve the patient's overall health, with a relief in migraines being a natural outcome of the treatment along with other positive side effects.

In Chinese Medical terms, migraines of an external origin occur when Wind-Heat, Wind-Cold or Wind-Damp invade the acupuncture channels located in the head. These are common syndromes, describing the process whereby environmental pathogens penetrate the body and impede the movement of blood and Qi (together referred to as lifeblood) to the head.

Internal causes include genetics, improper diet, emotional problems or chronic conditions caused by functional disorders of the Liver, Spleen or Kidneys. For example, a deficiency in the lifeblood can lead to malnourishment of the sensitive acupuncture channels in the head, which in turn causes migraine pain.
Another common syndrome recognised in Chinese Medicine as a root cause of migraine is a combination of internal Wind, build-up of phlegm and stagnation in the circulation of lifeblood, which

collectively cause blockages in the Shao Yang and Tai Yang acupuncture channels and lead to head pain.

Depending on the syndrome whereby the migraine has developed and the type of its cause (internal or external) identified by means of a detailed diagnosis, suitable Chinese herbs and acupuncture points are selected to treat the migraine at its root.

9) Chinese Medicine for Migraines related to Hormone Levels

Chinese Medicine combines herbal medicine and syndrome acupuncture to treat hormone-related migraines by subtly regulating the functional state of the Kidneys and the Liver – organs which both secrete hormones.
According to Chinese medical theory, Kidneys store the body's essential energy (a matter which is vital for sexual activity and reproductive health) and control the production of bone marrow. The Yang (hot) energy utilised by the Kidneys to support the body, and which is carried throughout the organism by the bloodstream, is also important for the nourishment of the brain. A lack of supply in such energy to the head typically causes migraine pain.
In the case of Kidney Yang deficiency, Chinese Medicine is used to tonify the Kidneys – particularly in relation to the Yang arm of the organ's operations – and ensure that the blood is circulating properly throughout the body so that the Yang energy is delivered to the head, brain is nourished and pain is alleviated through improved lifeblood circulation.
The Liver stores the blood (and therefore supports menstruation in women) and regulates the circulation of essential energy carried by the blood throughout the body. By using suitable Chinese herbs and stimulating the relevant acupuncture points Chinese Medicine can tonify the Kidneys, the Liver and subtly

Chapter 5) The Hormone Link

regulate their production of hormones - which in turn can treat the related migraine at its root cause.

General Information about Common Risk Factors from the Perspective of Chinese Medicine

Migraines are commonly experienced but can also be related to a person's genetics. The condition tends to be up to 2-3 more common amongst women than men and is more likely to happen during the menstrual periods. Migraines tend to occur more frequently during hormonal changes taking place in the period when the human body is 15-20 years old. The incidence of hormone-related migraines decreases during pregnancy and after menopause.

Chapter 6) Other Causes of Head Pain

Sometimes other conditions can be mistaken for migraines, as they can cause some of the same symptoms. Some patients will be experiencing migraines, but might also have another condition that is giving similar symptoms, making it appear that their migraines are more frequent than they really are.

Some of the conditions listed below are often mistaken for migraines, and in some cases, the following conditions can also trigger migraines. As detailed in the following chapter, TMJ is one of the conditions that can cause migraine-like symptoms and trigger migraines.

This is why it is important to see a doctor/physician if you haven't already so that you can ensure you are getting the proper treatment for your symptoms.

Detailed in this section are some conditions that can mimic migraines and suggestions for their treatment.

1) Sinus Headaches

These types of headaches can seem similar to migraines as they can make a patient sensitive to light and some patients with sinus headaches will also experience nausea. Other symptoms of sinus headaches include feeling congested, dizziness and face pain. Sinus headaches can also lead to pain behind the eyes and a high temperature. If you feel congested then it is more likely that the problem is sinus related and if the symptoms are severe then it might be necessary to take a course of antibiotics to help eliminate any infection.

If the symptoms are moderate try using nasal sprays, but not for longer than seven days, inhale steam or use a neti pot with a saline solution to help ease congestion.

Chapter 6) Other Causes of Head Pain

2) TMJ

TMJ can mimic the symptoms of migraines and it can also trigger an attack.

The symptoms of TMJ are a popping or clicking sound in the jaw, pain in and around the jaw, sensitivity to light and sound, muscle spasms in the upper body area and head pain, including migraines or just a general feeling of tension and pain in the head and face.

The symptoms of TMJ are pretty easy to spot, however, this is a condition that is often overlooked and patients with TMJ often get misdiagnosed.

If the migraines are worse in the morning or if you awake with pain in your head or face, then it is likely that TMJ is at least contributing to the migraines.

Treatment:

Like any other joint, the TMJ joint can become inflamed so an anti-inflammatory medication will often be prescribed in the early stages of the disorder.

Exercises are also useful to help improve the alignment of the jaw and massage will help to reduce the spasms,

Patients with TMJ should also avoid chewing gum and doing anything that puts an excess strain on the jaw joint.

When the pain is at its worse, give the jaw muscles a rest by eating softer foods such as soups and porridge – anything that doesn't involve using the jaw muscles too heavily when you eat.

3) Tension Type headaches

Tension type headaches are sometimes mistaken for migraines. Tension type headaches will often occur during a stressful period when a person is enduring a time in their life when they are experiencing a lot of anxiety or emotional stress.

These headaches can sometimes occur every day and leave a patient feeling as though they have constant head pain.

Treatment

In order to address the symptoms of tension type headaches, patients need to tackle the causes of them. If the headaches are caused by tension or stress then therapies such as CBT can be highly effective; osteopathy has also been shown to be useful. Tension type headaches can also develop when a patient has a lot of tension in their neck and shoulder region. This kind of tension is often caused by poor posture or activities such as typing or gaming.

4) Cluster Headaches

Often referred to as "suicide headaches" by their sufferers, cluster headaches are the most painful type of headaches. They occur in clusters and patients can be symptom free for month before suddenly experiencing a series of these excruciating headaches. Cluster headaches affect one side of the head and the pain is usually felt behind the eye. In some cases the eye can also become swollen or at least feels swollen.

Symptoms include a severe pain on one side of the head, watery eyes, a stuffy or running nose, sensitivity to light and sound and some patients can get an aura before an attack as well as nausea. In some cases, patients with cluster headaches will experience an increase in the blood pressure and in the heart rate.

Some of the triggers for cluster headaches are the same as with migraines; common triggers include strong scents, extreme weather conditions such as intense heat or cold, alcohol and spicy foods such as curry.

However, where cluster headaches differ from migraines is in their frequency and their intensity. While a migraine can last for a few days, cluster headaches can occur every day, several times a day, and the attacks can go on for weeks or sometimes months.

Treatment:

Treatment usually involves finding the right pain reliving medications to help manage attacks. Some of the medications that are prescribed for migraines are also often prescribed for cluster headaches.

Medications that might be suggested as treatment include Verapamil and triptan-based medications. Oxygen has also been shown to help manage cluster headaches.

Chapter 6) Other Causes of Head Pain

5) Rebound Headaches

Rebound headaches occur as a result of taking too much medication, Patients that take medications such as an anti-inflammatory drug or headache pills can find that they develop headaches when they are too dependent on pain killers.
Treatment:
By keeping a migraine or headache diary, it is easier to determine possible triggers. If the migraines occur more often when you are taking pain killing medication and you suspect that the medication is triggering the headaches, then this is something that should be discussed with your GP/Physician so that other medications can be prescribed.

Chapter 7) Coping With a Migraine

For many sufferers of migraines, it is not just the migraine itself that is the problem; it is coping with the symptoms that can occur before and after a migraine.
Managing migraines isn't just about treating the severe head pain, it is about finding all of the different ways to help manage the various symptoms such as feeling sick, sensitivity to light, and the over-tired, drained feeling that often comes with a migraine.
This chapter details some practical suggestions on how to cope with a migraine attack and some steps to take to help effectively manage them. There are also tips on how to reduce the feelings of nausea and managing light sensitivity.

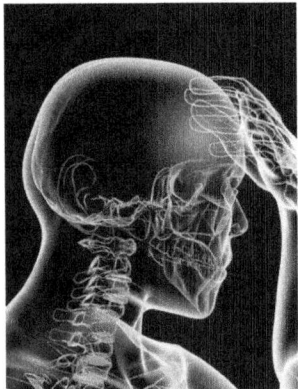

1) Rest
If possible, it is best to rest during and after a migraine as the attack can be very wearing on the body and some sufferers feel extremely tired after an attack.
If a patient has as sensitivity to light, then wearing an eye mask will help to keep out any light that might otherwise get into a darkened room.

2) Eat Regularly

Nausea and sickness will often leave a sufferer feeling as though they are unable to eat. However, proper nourishment is essential, especially if a person is feeling unwell following an attack.
Stick to light meals and eat them regularly to help keep the blood sugar level stable, as if the blood glucose falls too low, this can lead to a patient feeling drained as well.

3) Coping with Nausea

If the nausea is severe, then your doctor can prescribe medication, but there are some natural alternatives that can be tried. Here are some tips to help manage nausea.

a) Peppermint tea

Peppermint tea is well known to aid digestion and it can help to prevent nausea. The tea should not be drank while it is too hot and is usually best drunk when it has been left to cool for a while.

b) Ginger

Ginger is another helpful herb for managing sickness. It can be bought as a tea either on its own or as a combination with other herbs. Ginger can also be used as an essential oil or it can be brought in capsules or powder form.

c) Chamomile

The herb chamomile can help to stop nausea and it will also act to aid digestion and ease stress. As with other teas, it is best drank when it has been allowed to cool for a little while.

d) Fennel

Fennel tea helps to aid digestion and can help ease nausea. Prepare the tea as directed and drink it when it has been allowed to cool.
All of the herbs mentioned above can be brought as dried herbs and in capsule form as well.

Make any of the above teas up and sip them throughout the day in order to quell nausea and the digestive problems that can often result from a migraine.

If your temperature is high, then you can ice the teas and drink them cold.

e) Wristbands

Wristbands have been designed for travel sickness but they can also be used for other types of nausea such as that experienced by migraine sufferers.

4) Light Sensitivity

Even after the migraine has gone, light sensitivity can continue to be a problem making it difficult to look at the TV or computer monitor for long without it hurting the eyes.

To counter this, some people wear shades, but tinted lenses can also be extremely effective; opticians often suggest using a blue or yellow tint. Pin hole glasses can also be effective as they don't let in as much light and they are useful for avoiding eyestrain when watching the TV or looking at a computer screen.

If looking at a computer screen is difficult following an attack, either wear tinted glasses or get an anti-glare screen to go over the computer monitor. These are inexpensive to buy and they can be cut down to size to fit over any size computer screen so they are ideal for any monitor.

5) Manage muscle tension

For some patients, muscle tension can often be a factor in their migraines, and this is something that can be overlooked. Focus on reducing tension in the upper body area, concentrate on reducing stress in the upper body area such as the neck and shoulder. Neck spasm can be a common cause of migraine and reducing this tightness can help to reduce the number of attacks.

If neck spasms are known to be a problem with you, then you need to see a physiotherapist, an osteopath or a chiropractor to help reduce any accumulated tension.

6) Take things easy

It can be tempting to try and carry on as normal, but most migraine sufferers will realise soon enough that there just are times when they need to take things a bit easier and allow themselves to rest a bit more.

Make time for regular relaxation and ensure that you get at least six-eight hours sleep at night, especially if you have had a migraine recently as lack of sleep will contribute to headaches.

7) Find some balance

Everyone needs some balance in their life to help them to counter stress, but this is even more important for migraine sufferers. Stress is a common cause of migraines with some patients finding that stressful periods in their life can lead to more attacks, while other people find that it is after a stressful period has passed that they suddenly start to develop migraines.

Find ways to balance out your work life and leisure time and allow yourself enough time for yourself. In addition, don't allow yourself to feel pressurised into doing tasks or going to social events if you don't feel able to cope with them.

8) Forehead strips

Some patients notice an increase in temperature during an attack and these strips can help to lower the temperature and ease a headache in its early stages. These strips are also suggested as being suitable for migraine sufferers and they can help to relax the tense muscles in the forehead, so if muscle tension is a contributor to your migraines, then you might find these strips beneficial.

Massage balms are also useful for relaxing the temples, so if this is an area that you tend to gather tension, then a massage balm is useful to keep with you and they are small even to fit in a handbag or pocket.

9) Water

Dehydration can cause a migraine attack so keep the body hydrated by drinking plenty of water. Drinking still, un-carbonated water is by far the best way to keep the body hydrated and while the fluids contained within tea and coffee that might be drank throughout the day all count towards your fluid intake, they can also have a dehydrating effect.

If you are one of those people that just doesn't like the taste of tap water, then get a filter jug, and leave the water for a while before drinking it to give the chlorine taste time to fade. Store the water jug in the fridge so there is always some cold, fresh water to drink throughout the day.

10) Avoid excessive exercise

It can be tempting to push yourself a little harder when you are feeling good but excessive exercise that is extremely demanding on the body can contribute to migraines.

Many migraine sufferers will find that they will need to take life a little easier than others in order to avoid attacks, so don't try and keep up with everyone else.

If excessive exercise is a trigger for you, then find something that requires a much slower pace such as Hatha Yoga, Pilates or Tai Chi, or some light strength training to condition the muscles.

11) Use an ice pack

Some patients find that ice can help alleviate a migraine. Cooling eye masks are available. However, these aren't suitable for everyone, especially if a patient is cold intolerant or if they have sinus problems.

12) Heat

Some people tolerate heat much better than they tolerate cold. If a migraine has been caused by a muscle spasm in the neck area then using a heat pad on the back of the neck can help to relieve some of the tension.

Chapter 7) Coping With a Migraine

However, patients that have sensory problems such as the inability to feel heat should not use these.

13) Relax
Relaxation is vital for reducing the blood pressure and the heart rate. Take time out every day to do something to unwind. Choose from yoga, Tai Chi, Pilates, affirmations or meditation or anything else that helps to release stress and tension throughout the mind and body.

If you don't like any of the above activities then find something else to help you relax such as art or listening to music.

14) Keep a diary
Doctors often suggest keeping a diary to record migraine attacks. Sometimes the cause of a migraine might not seem obvious, but after keeping a record of events, medications, foods etc. it is much easier to find patterns and this will help you to discover the factors that can trigger a migraine, and will enable you to address the issues that have caused them.

15) Use an anti-glare screen
Some migraine patients find that they are more prone to migraines after spending a lot of time in front of the computer. Staring at a screen for long periods at a time is extremely taxing for the eyes and it can also place a strain on the neck; excessive neck tension is known to cause migraine in some patients.

If you are using a computer a lot, or if you use gadgets that require you to stare at a screen, then make sure that they are anti-glare, or that you buy an anti-glare screen to place over them.

This will reduce the amount of eye strain that occurs when staring at the screen for a long time.

Anti-glare screens are also useful for after a migraine as they help to reduce the uncomfortable feeling of the monitor screen looking too bright and hurting the eyes after an attack.

Chapter 7) Coping With a Migraine

16) Laptop stand

If neck tension is causing or contributing to your migraines, then try using a laptop stand if you do a lot of computer work; these are especially useful for netbooks as well.

Using a computer will often mean staring down at the screen, and for patients that are prone to migraines, then the neck tension that builds when staring down at a computer monitor or a netbook screen will make it worse, leading the way to more migraines. Make sure that the monitor is at eye level so that you don't need to look down at it; if you don't want to invest in a stand, then rest your netbook on a couple of sturdy books – anything so that the screen is at eye level and that you don't have to stare down for long periods at a time.

17) Get in touch with other sufferers

Some migraine sufferers can start to feel like that their migraines have taken over their life. Migraines can affect every aspect of a person's life from their ability to work if they are severe to the ability to socialise, which can mean a migraine sufferer will begin to feel isolated.

Other migraine sufferers can help by suggesting treatments and tips that they have tried themselves and speaking to other sufferers will help a migraine sufferer to realise that there are plenty of ways of effectively managing migraines.

Forums are useful; however, social media is playing an increasingly important part in allowing migraine sufferers to come together and share tips and advice.

There are many Facebook groups that are dedicated to migraine sufferers and there are a number of Twitter feeds as well. It is a good idea to take a look at these, and even if you don't feel like contributing or playing an active role, there is still the opportunity to learn from other people's experiences.

18) Caffeine

This doesn't work for everyone, however, some patients find that by taking their medication with caffeine, it will help it to get to

Chapter 7) Coping With a Migraine

work much quicker and many medications now contain caffeine for this reason. On the other hand, some patients find that caffeine will trigger a migraine or make it worse.

19) Find the right treatment

It might seem obvious, but once a patient has found the right medication or treatment, it can help change their lives. However, some patients will be prescribed a certain medication or will try an alternative therapy and because it doesn't work, they start to think that medication can't help them.

For many patients it can take several attempts until they get the right kind of medication to effectively treat their migraines. Everyone responds differently to medications, so what works for one person won't work for another and just because one person finds that their medication has changed their lives, it doesn't mean that it will work for you.

However, there are plenty of different types of medications, which give a patient plenty of opportunities to find something that works for them. Don't feel like you have to stick with just one form of medication; if your medication isn't working or if it gives you bad side effects, then speak to your doctor/physician and ask if you can try something else.

Likewise, some alternative therapies such as acupuncture or osteopathy work for some people. This will sometimes depend on what is causing the migraines. For instance, if muscle tension contributes to your migraines, then osteopathy is likely to be beneficial as it will help to reduce the tension and address any issues with your posture. Don't be scared of trying something different as once you have find the right treatment that works for you, then you won't look back.

Chapter 8) Stress Relief

1) Types of Stress

Stress is one of the common causes of migraines and as stated previously in the book, patients will often experience more migraine attacks when they are stressed or after a long period of stress.

Stress can be physical or emotional and can be major or minor. Examples of stress include:
- A house move
- Losing a job
- Illness
- Pain
- Losing a loved one

Stress has many negative effects on the body and can increase blood pressure, which can also leave a patient more prone to migraines. In addition, stress can cause blood sugar imbalance, insomnia and muscle tension, all factors that can increase the likelihood of a migraine.

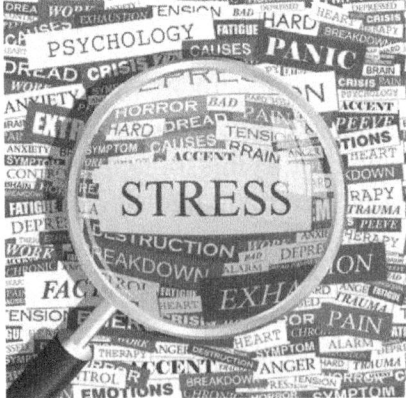

Another negative aspect of stress is that it will increase the cortisol levels. Cortisol is a hormone that the adrenal glands produce when the body is under stress.

Chapter 8) Stress Relief

Cortisol can be bad for the health for many reasons. First of all, it can cause a surge in the glucose levels and make the blood sugar much more difficult to control, it can cause difficulty sleeping and increase inflammation, which leaves the body more prone to pain and it will also increase the estrogen levels, which can leave a patient more prone to PMS.

While the body can effectively manage stressful periods for a while, there will eventually become a point where stress will begin to affect a person's overall well-being. Too much stress can leave a person feeling jaded and unable to cope with day to day life. This can eventually lead to burnout as the adrenal glands will eventually become exhausted.

The only real answer to this is to learn effective ways of managing stress. The most effective stress management techniques will be unique for everyone as everyone is different and everyone will have activities that they find enjoyable which others don't.

By finding stress management techniques and coping strategies, a person can learn to face their everyday challenges without feeling that it is all too much and like everything is too much effort or a constant struggle.

If you don't like the idea of some of the most popular relaxation techniques such as yoga, meditation or affirmations, then find an activity that you enjoy that will act as some form of release. It might just be listening to uplifting music, baking or art. It doesn't matter what it is, just find an activity that will help you to switch off from the everyday stresses of life and allow you to forget your problems for a while.

Marilyn Devonish is a Certified Master Practitioner and Trainer of Neuro Linguistic Programming (NLP), Certified Trainer of Hypnosis, Certified Trainer of Time Line Therapy, Certified PhotoReading and Accelerated Learning, and a Practitioner of various other modalities including EFT, Huna, Positive EFT,

Chapter 8) Stress Relief

Energetic NLP, DNA Theta Healing, EmoTrance, Soul Planning, and Archetypal Profiling.

In the next section, Marilyn Devonish explains some useful techniques for combating stress.

Stress in its purest form is almost the body being out of equilibrium and balance or being pushed beyond the limit of what the system feels it was designed to do. From the neurological perspective the sympathetic nervous system, the body's 'fight or flight' response is over stimulated, and is characterised by physical factors such as increased heart rate, constricted blood vessels and a rush of adrenalin. In psychological terms it can be characterised by emotions such as fear, anxiety, frustration, and anger.

Because of the arousal of the sympathetic nervous system, one of the first things that I would recommend when working with clients who don't respond well in stressful situations is to activate the parasympathetic nervous system, which is the body's natural relaxation response. The parasympathetic nervous system slows the heart rate, dilates the blood vessels, and allows for an increase in blood flow. This simple yet powerful exercise is a blend of what I teach my PhotoReading™ students, or running Presentation Skills Classes, both of which are environments that people tend to find highly stressful.

1. Take a deep breath in and exhale, and repeat this half a dozen or so times. This increases the oxygen flow around the body as well as sending a good supply of oxygen to stimulate the brain and help you think more clearly.
2. Get into peripheral vision or expanded awareness. When the body is under stress people automatically go into tunnel vision which starts to close down their awareness and focus in on the stressful situation and uses the more analytical part of the brain. Although great for those life threatening decisions, it is not so great for coming up with creative ideas or solutions because the right side of the brain takes a bit of a back seat.

Chapter 8) Stress Relief

Being in expanded awareness encourages left and right brain integration and enables clearer thinking and increases the likelihood of being able to come up with ideas or a solution. To check whether you are in peripheral vision, find a point to look at straight ahead, and whilst continuing to look straight ahead put your hands at either side of you head (much like you used to do as a child if you were going to stick your tongue out at someone) and then wiggle your fingers. If you can see your fingers moving without turning your head you are in peripheral vision. For those that are more into esoteric studies, in Hawaiian Huna terms, this is also referred to as the state of Hakalau, and is one of the Huna meditative practices.

3. Imagine a point located about 6 inches above and slightly behind the head and focus on that for a few moments. This helps to harness random thoughts and focus the mind. (This step is also a great process for those suffering with dyslexia, which in itself can be very stressful, particularly when people are attempting to keep it a secret).
4. As I noted earlier this relates to people who don't respond well in stressful situations. Stress and anxiety are also determined by our response to it, and the meaning that we assign. Some people often mistakenly see the stress as a source of fuel or internal motivation. This might be true in the short term, if however they don't have the capacity to deal with it, things can get out of control and it becomes a hindrance rather than a help.

2) NLP

There are several techniques from the field of NLP which are designed to help deal with stress and anxiety. A few of these include:

a) Changing the internal representation or Submodality

For example when I used to be terrified of spiders, and public speaking, the internal picture immediately invoked high levels of fear and stress. The picture in my mind was super large, I was seeing every awful moment and movement of those multiple legs through my own eyes, it was almost dark and muted with lots of lurking shadows, and there was a heaviness to it in the pit of the stomach, and a wave of panic that extended from the stomach through to the heart. An NLP Trainer or Practitioner would work with changing what are known as the Submodalies of the internal representation so that it no longer invokes an internal stress response, and mapping the old feelings across to the new state. The premise is that you think about the characteristics of something that you enjoy or find relaxing. The internal representation for the things that you enjoy will have key factors, which are vastly different to the first scenario.

b) Anchoring resourceful state
A popular methodology can be to anchor positive or resourceful states. The anchor can be a movement, a gesture, even a word which has associated to it how you want to respond instead. For example, in some sporting activities the competitors always enter the arena to a particular piece of music, which is an example of an anchor, something which invokes a state more conducive to the task in hand. Other people might have their lucky mascot or a gesture like punching the air and shouting 'yessss!'

c) Limiting beliefs
There can often be deeper underlying causes of stress and anxiety. Common beliefs that I encounter which limit a persons' ability to deal with a stressful situation include not being, or should I say not feeling, good enough, clever enough, capable enough, worthy enough. These beliefs act as filter through which people see the world and judge their performance or ability to perform in certain areas. For example when I held the belief that I wasn't good enough, my anxiety around public speaking was heightened because I began to question why anyone would even be remotely interested in what I had to say, and even if they were, I believed that I would more than likely have made a fool of myself. Unearthing and resolving these unhelpful beliefs gives a whole

new perspective on your ability to achieve things from a place of relaxation, ease and flow.

Identify the root cause. Aside from an array of techniques, of which there are hundreds I could choose from, one of the key things that I am interested in when working with a client is the root cause of the condition. From a therapeutic point of view, it might also be referred to that as 'secondary gain', meaning an underlying benefit of having things be this way. People will often initially object and can give 101 reasons why what they are experiencing is a problem and has no positive benefit or gain whatsoever. When you can identify the root cause of an issue and find a more ecological and healthy way to satisfy those needs, the stress response can disappear. For example I had a client who used to get the most terrible migraine headaches which of course seemed purely physical. The underlying secondary gain however was that the migraine meant they had to take some time out and have a rest, something which under normal circumstances they would rarely give themselves permission to do.

When we started identifying additional ways in which to take time out the migraines also started to disappear. The same is true for something like public speaking. The secondary gain might be to stop you from making a fool of yourself, so the mind and body will invoke a response to save you from this terrible fate. The resulting sabotage of course contributes to you falling into the very trap that you want to avoid, however that is not the first concern of the inner mind, whose primary function is to save you from the underlying apparent threat.

3) Chinese Medicine for Migraines related to Stress and Anxiety

In Chinese Medicine migraines linked to stress, anxiety and worry are associated with the Liver and the Heart. According to Chinese Medical theory problems such as anxiety, insomnia or too much stress trigger migraines because they impede the Liver's function of circulating lifeblood to the head, and, unsettle the Heart which is at the foundation of the person's mental state.

Stress can cause Fire (a kind of heat) within the Liver and unsettle the balance between the organ's cooling and warming properties, causing the latter (Yang, the opposite of Yin) to restlessly rise up the energy channel which links the Liver and the head and cause migraine pain. Insomnia and stress can also cause Fire within the Heart, which can have a knock-on effect on the supply of lifeblood to the brain and lead to head pain.

To alleviate migraine pain caused by stress, anxiety and/or insomnia, Chinese Medicine uses a combination of acupuncture and specific herbs to sooth the Liver and the Heart; clear out the Fire and control the rising Yang energy which, while relieving the patient's stress and improving their sleep, can alleviate the related migraine pains. By treating the patient's Liver and Heart with acupuncture and herbs, Chinese Medicine can strengthen the body's ability to cope with pain triggers such as stress and anxiety and hence lower the incidence of migraines.

It is also important to mention that, since migraines of internal cause are linked to diet in cases where certain foods trigger the symptoms, Chinese Medicine has identified the Spleen as a key organ in the diagnosis and formulation of treatment. In Chinese Medical theory the Spleen performs a major role in the digestive system as the organ, which processes the food and drink intake and assimilates the nutrients into the body.

Hence, Chinese Medicine states that in certain cases treatment of migraine must include regulating the functional state of the Spleen in order to improve the patient's ability to digest and absorb the foods which trigger the migraine symptoms.

4) Examples of Chinese Medicine Treatment Benefiting Patients with Migraines, at the AcuMedic Clinic

- A patient who was suffering from daily Migraine, had treatment involving acupuncture and massage at AcuMedic. The Migraine ceased after four treatments. One year later they had the same treatment to alleviate headaches (not Migraine). The result was a 90 percent improvement (with the addition of Herbal Tonic).
- "I was suffering from strong migraines during periods and repeatedly after. My previous treatments at AcuMedic were general for immune system and cosmetic acupuncture. My current treatments are the same plus I followed the advice and I am now having an amazingly efficient massage and the cupping. I feel extremely relaxed, happy no back or tension pain anymore."
"Acupuncture has helped relieve the symptoms of my migraine together with prescribed herbs."

5) Beating stress with diet

Diet is also an important way to help the body and mind to manage stress and the foods we eat can often leave us feeling jittery and anxious. Detailed below is a seven day eating plan to help aid stress management.

The following plan has been written based on a 25-35 year-old-woman, with an average height and weight, so adjust the servings accordingly, and if any of the foods suggested act as triggers, then find an alternative.

7 Day Plan for Helping reduce stress

Carbohydrates increase levels of serotonin, an anti-stress hormone. Complex carbs such as wholegrain cereals and bread will ensure a steady supply of serotonin. Treat yourself to simple carbs such as sweets and sugary drinks in moderation

Vitamins B and C are very important in managing stress, so eat plenty of apples for B vitamins, and citrus fruits for vitamin C

High magnesium foods, such as spinach, will reduce headaches and fatigue, and therefore stress.

The things to avoid most are cholesterol, salt and saturated fats, they will increase blood pressure and contribute to stress
Avoid coffee, worship tea (not herbal teas), and drink plenty of water.
Don't feel the need to stick to the order of this plan, think of the days more as options, mix and match it but keep the meals to their order.

Day One
Breakfast
Medium bowl of wholegrain cereal
1 Apple
Orange Juice
Lunch
Avocado, Lettuce and Tomato sandwiches with reduced fat mayonnaise and Swiss cheese

Evening Meal
Pasta with chilli, tomatoes and spinach

Day Two
Breakfast
Medium bowl of whole oatmeal
1 Apple
Orange Juice
Lunch
Spinach soup
Bread roll/bun
Evening Meal
Salmon steak
Boiled new potatoes
Green veg assortment
Raw salad items

Day Three
Breakfast
Apple, Orange and Banana chopped with granola and natural yoghurt
Lunch
Tuna + reduced fat mayonnaise sandwiches
Raw salad items
Evening Meal
Sweet Potato and Spinach bake (find recipes online)
Raw salad items

Day Four
Breakfast
Choose from previous options
Lunch
Chicken tikka sandwiches
Raw salad items
Evening Meal
Homemade Turkey burgers and Avocado fries (find recipes online)

Day Five
Breakfast
Choose from previous options
Lunch
Grilled chicken breast salad with kale, avocado and mango
Garlic bread
Evening Meal
Lightly breaded cod
Mashed potato (could mix with sweet potato)
Green veg assortment

Day Six
Breakfast
Choose from previous options
Lunch
Spinach and Feta pie
Raw salad items
Evening Meal
Sushi (with seaweed)

Day Seven
Breakfast
Choose from previous options
Lunch
Salmon sandwiches
Raw salad items
Evening Meal
Chicken/Turkey Sagwalla (curry with spinach)
Brown Basmati rice

Chapter 9) Blood Sugar Control

1) Low Blood Sugar and Migraine

Some patients find that they are much more prone to migraine when they are having problems controlling their blood sugar. Most often, people will find that when they go a long time without eating or skipping meals then they are more prone to low blood sugar levels.

A low glucose level will leave a person feeling jittery and stressed and when a person is feeling stressed, then more often than not they will turn to sugary foods to provide them with a quick boost. This only adds to the blood sugar imbalance and will make the glucose levels even more difficult to control.

Controlling the glucose levels will nearly always come down to what you eat, however, patients also need to be aware that stress can cause blood sugar problems and hormone imbalance can also influence the glucose levels causing them to run too high or too low. Balancing the blood sugars should concentrate on the following:

- Avoiding excess sugar
- Stress reduction and avoiding stressors
- Improving hormone balance

2) Avoiding Excess sugar

Excess sugar will increase the estrogen levels, making the blood sugars harder to control and causing a hormone imbalance that can leave women more vulnerable to migraines.

While avoiding the high-sugar snacks is easy enough for most people, many consumers will be alarmed at the amount of sugar added to pre-packed foods that are sold as healthier alternatives. Many convenience foods are loaded with sugar and are often high in salt, too; foods that are labelled as healthy are quite often high

Chapter 9) Blood Sugar Control

in sugar and contain several different types of sugar, all of which will contribute to a blood sugar imbalance as well as hormonal problems.

The healthiest thing to do is to prepare your own foods. Many people loathe to do this because of time constraints, but with some planning and some bulk cooking, preparing quick, healthy meals needn't take up too much time, and you'll always have a freezer full when you want something quick to eat.

For instance, making your own soups is quick and easy. They make a much healthier alternative to tinned soups and there is no sugar added. Soup recipes can be cooked in batches and frozen so there is always a quick meal ready for another day.

Likewise, meals containing pasta, whole grain rice, stews, casseroles etc., can all be cooked in bulk and frozen. This saves both time and money and will help you to avoid some of the sugar that is often added to meals.

White flour should also be avoided. Foods made with white flour will cause the blood sugars to soar in the same way that high sugar foods will. Avoid eating excessive amounts of white bread or breaded products as often as you can and this will help you to gain better control over your glucose levels.

3) Stressors

Stress can make it extremely hard to control the blood sugar levels. People that suffer from anxiety have a tendency towards low blood sugar, which can leave them feeling jaded and even more vulnerable to stress.

People that tend to get worked up easily, or find that are almost always in conflict with other people, and often get into arguments will find that they have a tendency to high blood sugars, which can be extremely damaging to health.

4) Diet

Diet is crucial for helping to maintain well-balanced blood sugar levels. A balanced diet won't just help with migraines, but it will also help to improve moods and improve energy.

5) Hypoglycaemia (Low Blood Sugar) Diet Plan

The Following diet plan has been drawn up by personal trainer Harvey B.

Eat every 3 hours during the day, in small meals to prevent spikes of blood sugar
Avoid caffeine
Avoid foods and drinks with high sugar levels, a sudden rise in blood sugar can cause hypoglycaemic reactions
Consume alcohol moderately
The plan below contains carbohydrates with a low glycemic index, foods with high fibre and plenty of protein.

Day One
Breakfast
Poached egg
Whole grain pumpernickel bread
Peach
Low fat milk or soy beverage
Lunch:
Wholemeal pitta
Sliced chicken breast and sweetcorn kernels
Reduced-fat mayonnaise
Dijon mustard
Lemon juice
Raw salad items
Snack:
Handful of plain nuts
Evening Meal:
Medium portion very lean Roast Beef
1 medium Sweet Potato roasted
Large portion Cabbage or Kale
Peas

Horseradish sauce.

Day Two
Breakfast
Oatmeal with ground flax seed, pecans and cinnamon
Blueberries or diced apples
Low fat milk
Water, or decaffeinated coffee or tea
Lunch
Medium portion of baked beans in tomato sauce
Large slice of wholegrain toast
Orange
Snack
Reduced fat hummus and 1 rye crisp bread
Evening Meal
Medium grilled Salmon Steak
1tbsp green Pesto sauce
Broccoli
Green beans
Medium portion of New Potatoes

Day 3
Breakfast
Traditional porridge made with skimmed milk
1tsp Honey
Orange
Lunch
Medium portion Brie
Cherry tomatoes
Spring onions and green salad leaves
1tbsp of olive oil vinaigrette
2 unsweetened rough oatcakes
Snack
Pear and a handful of pumpkin seeds

Chapter 9) Blood Sugar Control

Evening Meal
Medium portion falafel patties
Large stir-fry of sliced red peppers, red onion, tomato and courgette cooked in a little olive oil on a medium portion of bulgur wheat

Day Four
Breakfast
Large portion of low-fat bio yogurt mixed
1 chopped Apple and several chopped ready-to-eat dried Apricots
1 tbsp All Bran
1tsp Honey
Lunch
Medium portion Brie
Cherry tomatoes
Spring onions and green salad leaves
1tbsp of olive oil vinaigrette
2 unsweetened rough oatcakes
Snack
Pear and a handful of pumpkin seeds
Evening Meal
Large portion of grilled halibut, cod or other white fish steak,
1tbsp chilli tomato sauce
Petit pois
New potatoes

Day Five
Breakfast
Traditional porridge made with milk
Honey
Orange
Lunch
Large bowlful chilled vegetable and bean soup of choice
Medium slice Pumpernickel bread
Apple

Snack
1 pot low-fat fromage frais
Evening Meal
Large portion of grilled halibut, cod or other white fish steak, 1tbsp chilli tomato sauce
Petit pois
New potatoes
Grilled Tomato halves

The above diet plan has been written for females aged between 25-35, medium weight and a medium height. If you need to adjust the plan accordingly, then do.

Chapter 10) Stretching, Yoga and Meditation

1) Yoga

As previously discussed, migraines can sometimes result from tension in the neck muscles. Moreover, people who find that they get stressed easily are also more likely to develop migraines. Mental stress will often lead to physical tension so learning to relax is essential for helping to reduce migraines.

This chapter focuses on yoga stretches and exercises that are designed to reduce tension in the upper body, relax the mind, and to help ease anxiety.

The exercises should be carried out in a warm, quiet place; wear loose clothing for comfort and make sure that you won't be disturbed. These exercises are best carried out last thing at night, but can be used whenever you feel stressed or if you feel that the muscles in the upper body are tightening up.

The first part of this chapter details some yoga exercises and the second part details stretches. These exercises can easily be integrated into the day and you could also practice the exercises on alternate days i.e. yoga one day and the stretches the next if you don't have time to complete the entire routine every day. Some patients find that they experience headaches when doing forward bend postures, however, this is often due to the way that the postures are carried out and not due to the posture themselves.

a) Child's Pose

This yoga pose is one of the most effective for reducing the tension that accumulates in the upper back and in between the shoulder blades. Tension that accumulates in this area can cause excess tightness in the neck muscles that can ultimately lead to a neck spasm; a neck spasm can cause migraine in some people Child's pose will also stretch the legs, ankles and knees.

Precautions:
Patients with blood pressure problems should be careful with this posture. People with knee or ankle problems/pain should also take care.

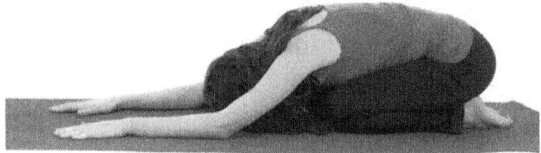

Directions:
Using a mat or a soft surface, kneel with the toes together and sit up straight in preparation for the move. Take a breath outwards and as you do, move forward so that your torso rests on your knees.
This move can be held for as long as is comfortable, however, be careful not to hold the move too long as it can sometimes cause a spasm in the lower legs

b) Forward Bend

Forward bend postures are ideal postures for quietening the mind and reducing anxiety. They can be performed whenever you have a quiet moment or whenever you feel that your mind is racing and you want something to help slow your thoughts down.

They are good for practising throughout the day if the opportunity arises, as the posture will also help to make you feel focused, refreshed, and ready for the rest of the day. Forward bend postures also help to stretch the legs and reduce tension in the lower back.

Don't practice this posture if you feel at all unwell or if you have had a migraine recently.

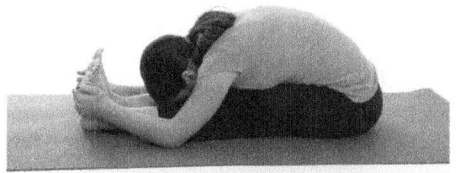

Directions:

Sit up straight on a yoga mat or soft surface. Make sure that your spine is straight and that your legs are together and stretched out in front of you. As you exhale, reach out and take hold of your feet with your hands.

Your hands can either grasp your feet at the ankles or the toes; if you have limited flexibility then reach to the shins. You can also use a belt or exercise band to stretch into this posture.

Lower your head so it is as close to your knees as possible, keeping the breath steady throughout the posture.

Hold the posture for up to five breaths or 30 seconds.

Precautions:

Patients with lower back, leg and shoulder problems should take care with this posture. Patients with blood pressure problems should also be careful with this posture.

Don't practice this posture if you have just had a meal and don't practice this posture if you are feeling at all unwell.

c) Warrior Pose

Warrior poses are an energetic set of postures that can leave you feeling positive and energised. They are good for practicing when you have a long day and you need an energy boost.

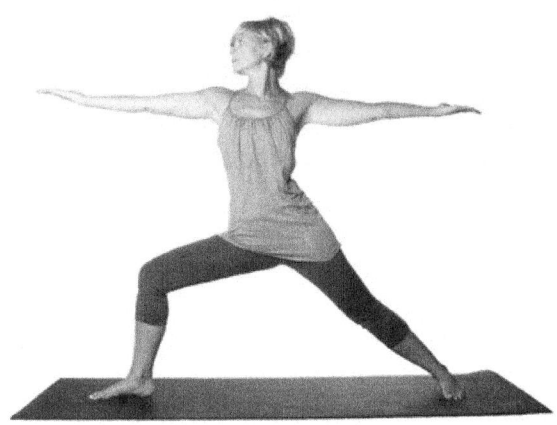

This pose helps to open up the neck, shoulders and upper back area; it is also an ideal stretch for opening up the chest muscles, which often become tight when we are sat cramped over a computer or when we do repetitive tasks.

Directions:

Breathe out, and on the exhale, jump or step your feet until they are three-four foot apart. Turn the left foot out to a 45 degree angle and the right foot should be pointing forwards at a 90 degree angle.

Twist your torso so that your are facing forwards and bend your right knee; make sure that your knee does not reach out over your foot or you'll put too much stress on the joint.

Raise your arms until they are parallel and keep the gaze outwards. Hold the posture for five breaths.

Precautions:

Patients with heart conditions or high blood pressure should not attempt this move. Patients with neck problems might feel pain if they look up at their hands, so should keep their gaze forward and stare outwards rather than up at the hands.

d) Standing Forward Bend

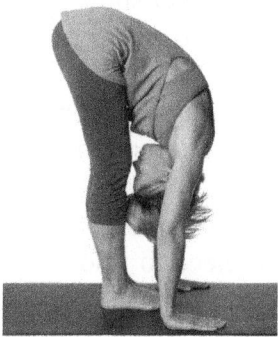

Directions:
Reach your arms up above your head and then slowly fold forward until your head rests on your knees and either reach your hands to the floor or reach your hands to just above your ankles and gently grasp them. If you are unable to reach your ankles or the floor then just reach to the shins.. Hold the posture for five breaths

This is an excellent posture for calming the mind and relaxing the upper body. Be careful when moving into this posture as it can leave you feeling light headed if you move into it too quickly. Also, be careful when coming out of the standing forward bends, as this can also cause light headedness

Precautions:
This pose shouldn't be practiced by people with blood pressure problems. Patients with headaches should take extra care when carrying out this posture and patients with tight hamstrings or a hamstring injury should be careful with this posture.

All of the forward bend postures in yoga can be beneficial for calming the mind and reducing stress and anxiety, so these can be practiced on a regular basis if they are found to be beneficial. However, some people find that they develop headaches while in forward bends. This is not usually because of the posture itself, but because of the way the pose is performed.

Chapter 10) Stretching, Yoga and Mediation

If you are in any doubt over the forward bend postures and whether they are right for your circumstances, then get some advice from a yoga teacher before doing any of the forward bend postures detailed in the book.

If you are feeling at all unwell, have had a recent migraine, or feel as though you have a migraine coming on, do not attempt any of these postures as they could make you feel worse.

However, you might find the meditation or visualisation beneficial if you are feeling unwell or tense and need to find an effective way to unwind.

A creative visualisation and a meditation have been included later on in this chapter and can be recorded and listened to whenever you feel the need as you go about your day or it can used for a relaxation aid last thing at night.

e) Triangle Pose

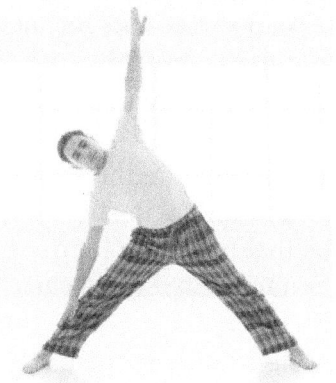

The triangle pose provides a great stretch for the legs and lower body, however, it can also provide a powerful stretch for the shoulder area and it is useful for reducing tension in the shoulder region.

Directions:
Step or jump your feet until they are 3-4 feet apart; keep your stance narrower if you find it difficult to balance. Slide your right hand down your right side until it reaches the ankle and extend your left hand up. If you are unable to reach the ankle, then stretch to the shin.

Next, either look up towards your hand, or if you have a neck problem, keep the gaze outwards. Hold the posture for five rounds of breath and then slowly come out of the pose.

Precautions:
People that suffer from headaches or migraines need to take care with this pose, however, when practised carefully this posture should not cause any problems. If you are not sure about this posture, then it is best to take the advice of a yoga instructor who can discuss modifications with you.

Patients with neck problems should also take care with this posture, as should patients with a back problem.

Chapter 10) Stretching, Yoga and Mediation

2) Stretches

Reducing stress in the neck and shoulder area can be extremely beneficial to migraine sufferers. Migraines can sometimes be due to excess tension in the neck muscles so regularly stretching of the muscles in this area will be most beneficial to patients who have tight muscles in the neck.

The following stretches will help to reduce tightness in the neck and shoulder area. They will help prevent neck and pain shoulder from developing and if you carry out tasks that involve a lot of repetitive stress on the upper body area then these exercises can be extremely beneficial.

The exercises will also help to reduce muscle tension in the chest area, which can help make the breathing more relaxed; which in turn can help to reduce stress.

a) Simple shoulder stretch

This stretch can be carried out at any time during the day. It is useful for people that find they tense up while they are working or if they are feeling stressed and it will help to free up the shoulder area.

Repeat this stretch as often as needed throughout the day.

Directions:

Interlink the hands and stretch them over head. Hold the pose for as long as is possible. The stretch should be felt in both shoulders and in the shoulder blades.

For a deeper stretch, ease the arms a little further back; stretch the arms towards the right if there is tightness in the right side or to the left to add an extra stretch for the left side.

b) Simple Neck Stretch

Computer users can gain a lot of benefit from carrying out this stretch regularly.

This neck stretch can be carried out while lying down or while sat at a desk or in a chair. To avoid injuring the neck, use small, gentle, slow movements.

Chapter 10) Stretching, Yoga and Mediation

Start at the centre and then simply turn the head to the left as far as it will go without causing strain or discomfort and then repeat to the right. Hold each stretch for about five seconds.

This exercise can also be carried out by resting the neck on a ball. To perform this exercise, you'll need a soft, medium sized ball, such as the ones that are often used in Pilates.

Directions:

Lie back on a bed with the neck resting on the exercise ball. Turn all of the way to the left, keeping the movements smooth, and without jerking, and return to the centre. Repeat on the right side.

c) Shoulder Stretch

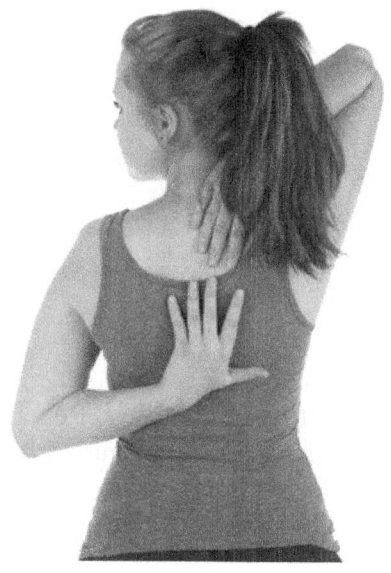

This stretch will help to loosen up the shoulder region while helping to improve flexibility. Depending on how tight the arms arm, some people might not be able to interlink their fingers. If this is the case, use an exercise band or belt until the shoulders become more flexible.

Directions:

Place the right hand face down in between the shoulder blades. Bring the left hand behind you and walk the fingers of the left hand up your back as far as you can comfortably go. The aim is to

get the fingers of both hands so that they are interlinked, but many people are not able to do this to begin with.
With regular practice, it will eventually become possible to link both hands, which is a positive sign that the shoulder area is beginning to loosen up.

d) Shoulder Stretch 2

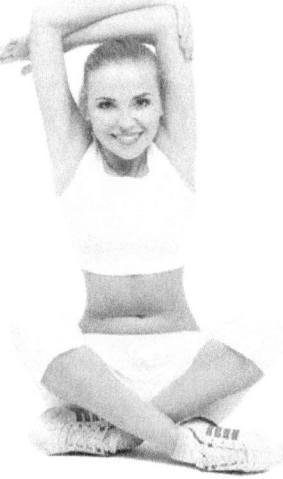

This exercise can be performed either sitting or standing. Reach one arm so that it rests on the top of the head; don't use any pressure. Reach your other arm up until your hand touches on the elbow and hold the position until you feel a gentle stretch in the shoulder.

e) Shoulder Stretch 3

Reach your left hand behind you so that it touches in between the shoulder blades. Bring up the opposite hand so that it touches the elbow and apply some gentle pressure on the elbow joint until you feel a stretch in the shoulder.

Chapter 10) Stretching, Yoga and Mediation

3) Meditation

A meditation session can be carried out before or after the stretches and yoga poses. Some people prefer to meditate before they begin yoga as it helps to calm the mind, however, some people prefer to meditate afterwards as the yoga will have already quietened the mind, and with the mind quiet it is easier to focus on the meditation.

There is no "best time" for doing meditation, find a time that suits you the best. For some this will be in the morning to help achieve a calm, focused mind, for others it will be last thing at night. Meditation doesn't have to be complicated, just closing the eyes and counting the breath is enough. Detailed below is simple meditation along with a creative visualisation.

a) Meditation

This meditation is ideal for carrying out at the end of a long day, but is can be used whenever you feel the need to relax.

Directions:

Sit in a cross legged position, or sit up straight with your hands on your knees, whichever is the most comfortable.

Shut your eyes and take a few moments to clear your mind of any thoughts. Don't worry if you continue to get intrusive thoughts as you practice the meditation; this will happen less often the more you practice.

Focus on your breath. If your breathing is fast, concentrate on slowing it down. Slowly count every inhale and exhale until you feel your mind calming down and your breath slowing.

When your breath is calm, create an image in your mind. The image can be anything you want it to be- a dream island, a candle, a heart, choose anything that is significant to you and that helps you to feel more relaxed.

Alternatively, picture a safe place. It might be a place that you used to go to as a child where you always felt calm and happy.

Chapter 10) Stretching, Yoga and Mediation

Don't think of anything else, if your mind does wander – and it often does during meditation – then bring the focus back to your object.

Try and stay in this meditation until your mind goes completely still and then slowly open your eyes.

When the meditation is complete, take a few more minutes to concentrate on your breath.

b) Relaxing Visualisation

Visualisation is perfect for helping you to feel however it is you want to feel. If your mood needs a boost, simply picture happy, positive scenes in your mind or if you feel stressed, picture relaxing, calming images.

Lie back on a bed or use a yoga mat/blanket or lie on the floor if you need a firmer surface.

Close your eyes and picture yourself walking towards your favourite, relaxing destination. It might be a day at the beach or in the forest, just think of the place that you love the most.

Picture yourself taking slow, meaningful steps, and with every single step you take imagine yourself getting closer to your destination. Count the steps if it makes relaxation easier.

Continue this until you are feeling relaxed and calm and the breath has slowed.

Once you have reached your destination, picture a place where no one else can find you – a place only you know. It doesn't have to be a real place, just picture somewhere that is for you and you alone.

Picture yourself in this place with no one to bother you, and no sound around you, except the natural sounds of the environment; a place of perfect peace.

Stay there in your mind, in your safe place, until your mind becomes perfectly relaxed and still and the body feels ready for sleep.

Chapter 11) Recipes

Enhancing the serotonin levels, evening out the blood sugars or providing essential nutrients such as magnesium to help manage migraines.
Each recipe serves 2-4 people and many of them can be made ahead or cooked in bulk and frozen so there is always something ready to eat if you need a healthy meal and don't have time to cook or prepare something from scratch.
If any of the ingredients listed are a trigger for you or if you don't like any of the ingredients, then substitute them with something else.

1) Goats Cheese Salad

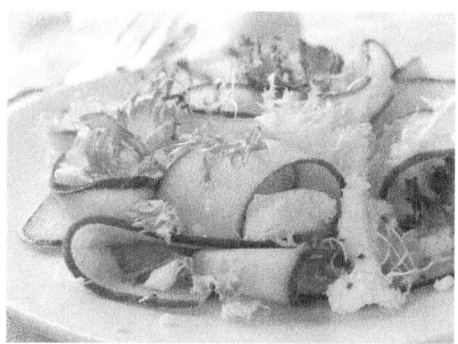

As many people find cheeses a trigger for their migraines, this recipe uses goat's cheese as an alternative. The green vegetables supply essential nutrients such as magnesium and Vitamin C.
Ingredients:
Iceberg Lettuce
Half a Cucumber
8 – 10 cherry tomatoes
Half a red pepper

Half a green pepper
Goats cheese (6-8 slices)
Seeds such as sunflower seeds or pumpkin seeds
Oil
Directions:
Begin by washing all of the vegetables under cold water.
Cut an iceberg lettuce into quarter and shred or tear the leave or use a bag of ready prepared ice burg. Arrange them on a plate, cut the cucumber into thin slices and slice and dice the peppers. Add these to the plate and then add the cherry tomatoes.
Scatter the seeds over the salad and then add a light drizzle of oil. Choose any kind of oil and then add the goat's cheese.
Serve with a granary roll.
The recipe is enough to serve two people.

Chapter 11) Recipes

2) Carrot and Parsnip Soup

This quick soup can be made in a large quantity and frozen in individual portions. It keeps well in the freezer for several months.

Ingredients:

Two large carrots, sliced
One large parsnip, sliced
Half an onion, sliced
One pint of vegetable stock
Herbs of choice (coriander works well)

Directions:

Either use a ready prepared stock or make your own by boiling the ends of chopped vegetables in water and then strain it once it has cooled.

Wash the vegetables and slice or dice them.

Add the stock to the saucepan, followed by the vegetables. Leave to cook cooking on a medium heat until the vegetables are soft, but still have some texture.

Allow to cool for a while before serving in soup plates.

This recipe serves two, and can also be blended if it is preferred. Serve with a granary or wholemeal roll.

Chapter 11) Recipes

3) Quinoa, Courgette and Carrot Stew

This recipe cooks well in a slow cooker, so can be prepared ahead of time. It can also be served cold for lunch the next day and it keeps well in the fridge for a few days.

Ingredients:
One courgette, sliced
One – two carrots, sliced
Half an onion, sliced
Tinned tomatoes
Vegetable stock
One packet of quinoa

Directions:
Prepare the vegetable stock according to the directions; allow to cool.
Prepare the quinoa according to the directions on the packet.
Wash the vegetables and then slice them.
Add the stock to the slow cooker and then add the quinoa gradually and vegetables. If it looks like too much, then just use half of the quinoa.
Pour over the tinned tomatoes and stir everything together so that there is a good mix of vegetables.
Leave to cook on a medium heat. This usually takes approximately two hours, but will vary according to the different models.

Chapter 11) Recipes

4) Tomato and bean Soup

Beans provide phytoestrogens that are helpful in balancing out the hormone levels and tomatoes contain vitamin C, which is good for supporting the adrenal glands, thus helping the body to cope better with stress.

Ingredients:
Pulses (choose from kidney, butter beans, chick peas, mixed beans and use tinned beans for quickness)
One pint of vegetable stock (either homemade or shop brought)
Half an onion, chopped
Six large tomatoes

Directions:
Wash the tomatoes and then blend them one at a time.
Prepare the vegetable stock and add it to a large saucepan.
Next, add in the blended tomatoes and stir. Add the onion; stir.
Mix in the pulses (One - two tins should be plenty as they are extremely filling)
Simmer on a low heat until the ingredients are hot all of the way through.
Serve with a green salad of lettuce, cucumber, pepper and celery or with a granary or wholemeal roll.

Chapter 11) Recipes

5) Tuna and Pasta B

Pasta is rich in B vitamins and tuna contains Omega 3 oils. Omega oils help to lift the mood, helping to reduce stress and anxiety.

Ingredients:
One large tin of tuna fish, drained, if using tuna in oil, ensure that it drained properly first.
One tin of tomatoes (chopped)
500 grams of wholemeal pasta
Half an onion, chopped

Directions:
Cook the pasta in accordance with the directions on the packet.
Make a quick pasta sauce by combining the tinned tomatoes with the chopped onion or use a low sugar ready-made pasta sauce.
Add the pasta to an oven dish. Pour over the tomato sauce.
Mix in the tinned tuna and combine all of the ingredients well.
Allow to cook until it is hot all of the way through.
For a variety, add in broccoli or sweetcorn into the bake.

Chapter 11) Recipes

6) Barley and Vegetable Casserole

Barley is an often under used cooking ingredient, but it is cheap and filling and packed full of B vitamins. Barley is also a low glycaemic food so it is ideal for balancing out the blood sugar levels.

The casserole freezes well and will keep up to three months, so this is an ideal recipe for cooking in bulk.

Ingredients:
One packet of no soak barley
Two large carrots, sliced
Two celery stalks, sliced
One onion, sliced
One pint of vegetable stock

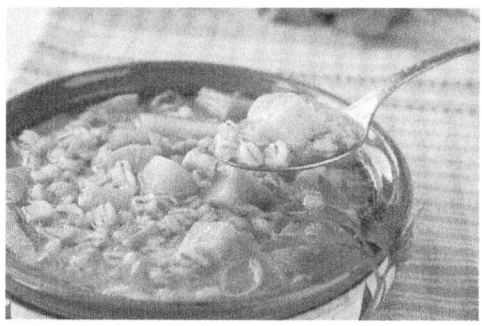

Directions:
Wash and slice all of the vegetables.
Make up the stock according to the directions, or use a home-made stock and add it to a large pan. Add in the barley and allow to cook. Barley can take one – one and a half hours to cook and it needs to be cooked through properly. Cook the barley on a low heat.
Keep checking that the liquid doesn't run too low. If it does, prepare more stock, or add some water.

While the barley is cooking, wash and slice the vegetables.
With the barley almost cooked, add in the vegetables (they'll need to go in approximately 10-15 minutes before end of cooking time)
Allow to simmer until all of the ingredients are cooked through.
Allow to cool for a short while before serving.
To add some more flavour use leeks instead of celery and blend in tinned tomatoes or fresh, blended tomatoes.

7) Turkey Stir Fry

Turkey contains tryptophan, an amino acid that helps us to feel relaxed and calm and the vegetables add important vitamins and minerals.

Ingredients:
One packet of diced turkey pieces
One packet of bean sprouts
Red, green, or yellow pepper
One red onion, sliced
6- 10 mushrooms, sliced or buy ready sliced mushrooms, and use half of the packet
One celery stalk, sliced
Olive oil or sunflower oil for cooking

Directions:
Add 2-4 tablespoons of oil to the frying pan; warm the frying pan on medium heat.
Begin by cooking the turkey meat.
While the meat is gently cooking through, wash and slice the vegetables and add them to the pan along with the beansprouts. Turn the ingredients over regularly so that they get a coating of oil and don't burn.
Once all of the ingredients have cooked through thoroughly, the stir fry is ready to serve.

Chapter 11) Recipes

8) Bean Bake

This unusual combination makes a filling, quick meal. If you don't like beans, then use wholemeal pasta.
This recipe includes pulses to stabilise the blood sugars and vegetables to for their vitamin and mineral content.
If cheese is a trigger for you, then use a non-dairy alternative.
Ingredients:
One tin of chopped tomatoes
Half a courgette, sliced
Half an onion, sliced
One tin of mixed beans, butter beans, chick peas or kidney beans
Grated cheese
Breadcrumbs
Directions:
Wash and chop the vegetables. Place the courgette in a saucepan to cook while you prepare the rest of the recipe.
Line an oven dish with foil and add the beans or pasta in the bottom.
Slice the onion; add half of it to the beans.
Add the cooked courgette and add it to the other ingredients.
Top with the tinned tomatoes and scatter enough grated cheese on top to cover all of the ingredients.
Sprinkle over the bread crumbs and leave to cook on a medium heat until it is hot all of the way through.

Chapter 11) Recipes

9) Green Salad

This salad is full of vital vitamins and minerals and it is quick to prepare.
Ingredients:
50 grams of rocket
75 grams of lettuce
Half a cucumber, sliced
One green pepper, sliced
1-2 celery stalks, sliced
Seeds
Directions:
Wash and slice the vegetables.
Add the lettuce to a plate and layer the rocket on top.
Add some oil. Blend it with some lemon juice if you want some added flavour.
Add the other vegetables to the plate and drizzle some more oil on the top.
Scatter with some seeds. Choose sunflower, sesame or pumpkin.
Serve with a wholemeal or granary roll, crisp breads, or oatcakes.
Alternatives:
If you don't like any of the ingredients included in the above recipes, then choose an alternative ingredient. Choose any green vegetables, as they are high in magnesium.

10) Mediterranean Pasta

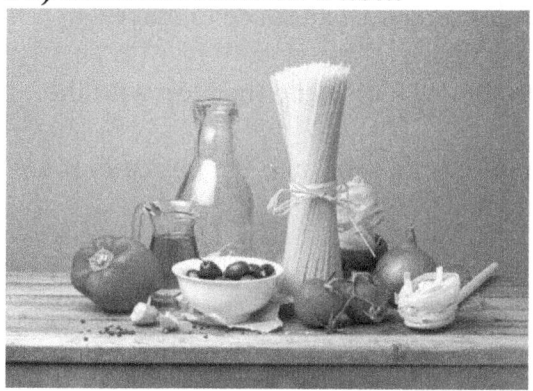

The Mediterranean diet is regarded as one of the healthiest in the world and includes plenty of vegetables, fruits, pulses, grains and oils.
This quick to prepare meal can be cooked in less than 30 minutes and makes a satisfying meal.

Ingredients:
500 grams of pasta (any variety)
One tin of tomatoes
One onion, red or brown, chopped
One red pepper, chopped
One courgette, chopped
A handful of olives
Drizzle of oil

Directions:
Prepare the pasta according to the instructions on the packet.
While the pasta is cooking, wash and chop the vegetables; cook the courgettes in the same pan as the pasta to speed up cooking time.
Lightly fry the onion.
Add the cooked pasta to an oven dish along with the courgette and some of the onion.

Chapter 11) Recipes

Add the other vegetables.

Make a quick pasta sauce by combining the tomatoes with the onion or use a ready-made, low sugar pasta sauce to make preparation time quicker.

Add the other vegetables to the oven dish and then top with the pasta sauce.

Bake for approximately 20-25 minutes or until the ingredients are cooked all of the way through.

Chapter 11) Recipes

11) Fish Pie

The potatoes contained in this recipe provide serotonin, which helps to calm the mind and reduce anxiety. Fish contains Omega 3, which can help to lift the mood.

Ingredients:
Two medium sized salmon fillets
Cheese sauce (Use a non-dairy alternative if cheese is one of your triggers).
Mashed potato
Breadcrumbs

Directions:
Cook the salmon on a medium heat until cooked all of the way through.
Cut the salmon into small pieces and add to an oven dish.
Make up a cheese sauce using a non-dairy alternative such as rice milk. Once the sauce has thickened enough, pour it over the salmon fillets. Add the mashed potato on top and sprinkle on a light coating of bread crumbs.
Allow to bake until it is hot all of the way through and the top is golden brown.
Serve with carrots, broccoli and cauliflower
To make the cheese sauce:
115gs of Grated Cheese
115gs of Flour
Quarter of a point of milk
Knob of butter

Directions:
Mix the cheese, half of the flour, the milk and the butter to a saucepan and warm on a medium heat. Add more flour as necessary to ensure that the sauce thickens.
Stir the ingredients until the sauce becomes thick and smooth.

12) Turkey Pie

The potatoes and turkey provide serotonin, which makes the mind feel calm.
This makes a quick, tasty meal. The surplus can be frozen; however, it will need extra stock when it comes to reheating it, as it tends to dry out if left to freeze for too long.

Ingredients:
450gs of turkey mince
Chicken or beef stock, or use beef or chicken gravy as an alternative.
Half an onion, chopped
Mashed Potato

Directions:
Fry the turkey mince on a medium heat until it is cooked all of the way through. Add the chopped onion to the frying pan and cook it until it is golden brown.
Add the turkey and onion to an oven dish that has been lined with silver foil.
Make up the stock or gravy according to the directions on the packet. You'll need just enough stock to flavour the meal, but don't add too much or the juices will run when it is served. If using gravy, make enough to form a thin layer over the turkey mince.
Add the stock/gravy.
Add the mashed potato and smooth is out over the top of the pie. Leave to cook until the ingredients are hot all of the way through and the topping is golden brown.
To make the mashed potato for the above two recipes follow these instructions:

Up to 500g of Potatoes, boiled

Pinch of salt

100ml of milk
Knob of butter
Mash the potato with the butter and stir in the milk. Add a little bit at a time so it doesn't get too runny.
At some seasoning such as salt and pepper if you wish.

13) Quick Snacks

Pita Bread pizza
This makes a healthy, fast alternative to pizza.
What you need:
One small, wholemeal pita bread
Grated cheese, or a dairy alternative if cheese is a trigger.
One large tomato, sliced
Half an onion, sliced
Any other vegetables/ toppings of choice.
Cover a pita bread with cheese, or dairy alternative.
Add the other ingredients.
Allow to cook under the grill, in a microwave, or in the oven under it is lightly brown all over.
Serve with a green salad.

14) Baked Sweet Potato

Baked Potatoes make a healthy snack and the sweet potato is an even healthier alternative as it is full of beta carotene, hence the orange flesh.
Slice a sweet potato down the middle and cook it in the microwave, or leave it to slow cook in the oven.
Serve with a topping of your choice and salad

Chapter 11) Recipes

15) Sweet Treats

Everyone likes to treat themselves now and again, however, if low blood sugar is a problem for you of if you have a hormone imbalance, then you'll want to stay away from the sweet stuff as often as you can.
That doesn't mean that it isn't OK to have the occasional sweet snack. However, when you want something sweet, have it with a main meal to help curb any swings in the blood sugar and make your own snacks so that you can ensure that they don't contain too much sugar.
Flapjack Recipe
Oats contain high levels of B vitamins so they are excellent for helping the body to cope with stress and anxiety. This recipe makes up to twelve bars.
Flapjacks make a great alternative to chocolate bars and the complex carbohydrates help even out any surge in the blood sugar levels.
These are great for snacks in the morning or afternoon and they also make a good dessert.
This recipe makes approximately 12 flapjacks and they will keep in an airtight tin for a week to ten days.

Ingredients:
500gs of rolled oats
250gs of margarine or butter
3-4 tablespoons of Golden Syrup- use more if the recipe doesn't bind together.

Dircctions:
Gently heat the margarine/butter in a saucepan
Mix in the rolled oats and stir them in well until they are all coated with the butter.

Chapter 11) Recipes

When the ingredients are fully combined, stir in the syrup. If 3-4 tablespoons isn't enough, then add some more until the whole mix holds together.

Add the mixture to a small, square oven dish and then leave to bake until golden brown.

Alternatives:

For flapjacks with a difference, add some pumpkin seeds, sesame seeds or sunflower seeds.

Chapter 11) Recipes

16) Fruit Salad

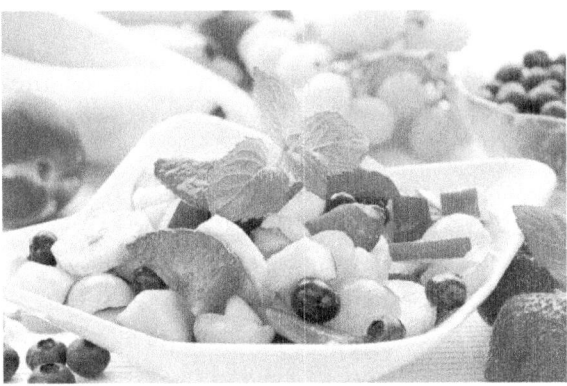

Fruits provide the body with important vitamins and nutrients and a fruit salad is a healthy alternative to most of the shop bought desserts that are available today.

You can combine any combination of fruits, but steer clear from fruits that contain fast releasing sugars such as bananas if you don't want any sudden spikes in your blood sugar.

If you want to prepare this recipe and eat it later, then add a small amount of lemon juice to stop it going brown.

Ingredients:
One apple, washed and sliced,
One pear, washed and sliced
One kiwi fruit, peeled and sliced
6-8 strawberries, washed and sliced
Two tablespoons of pineapple chunks, unsweetened.
If you don't like any of the above fruits, just replace them with another, but don't choose fruits with fast releasing sugars.

Directions:
Arrange all of the ingredients onto a plate and mix well so that there is a good blend of fruits.

Chapter 11) Recipes

Either serve on its own, add a small amount of honey, or unsweetened, organic, natural yoga.
Other Sweet Ideas:
Sugar Free Jelly with two tablespoons of organic, natural yogurt
Unsweetened pineapple junks served with organic, natural yogurt

17) In Between Meals

People often turn to junk food in between meals to give them energy, but the following foods provide a much healthier alternative,
- Crisp breads or oat cakes with hummus
- Porridge pots, unsweetened, or lightly sweetened
- Seeds
- Unsalted popcorn
- Fruit
- Pure fruit bars

Appendix One: Migraines, A Personal Experience

Here, one migraine sufferer shares their experience of migraines and suggestions for self- treatment:

Many treatments are recommended for migraine but there are various self-treatments that can be practiced. I had a severe migraine but now with treatment, I'm able to overcome the migraine and manage the symptoms. A proper rest and sleep is a preamble to migraine treatment. Any physical activity enhances the severity of headache, thus a break is needed.
Irregularity in my sleeping routine triggered migraine so I tried not to have too many late nights and slept at the same time every night; it lessened the headache. I also switch off the lights when I'm having migraine; it lessens the pain and relaxes my nerves. Temperature therapy is very effective and can be easily done. Using ice packs may dull the sensation by causing a numbing effect. Likewise, warm showers and baths can relax the tense muscles and lower the pain.

Massage is another way to get rid of pain, gently pressing the scalp relieves me of the pain. Caffeine is also effective too. In moderate amounts it can help in reducing the pain but a large amount of it can cause the headache, so be careful. A cup of coffee would be enough for most people. But for some people caffeine can be a trigger, so be watchful and identify your personal triggers.

Never miss your meals. Eat three times a day and stay healthy. Whenever my eating habits got disrupted, migraine attacks came back like devouring bats making me feel uneasy and tensed. So, I advise you to not to skip a meal and keep eating.

Appendix One: Migraines, A Personal Experience

As a Migraine sufferer I experience a symptom called an aura; it is a signal that migraine is going to occur. To tone down its effects, finding a dark place with lesser auditory, visual and olfactory stimuli is effective.

Essential oils can be massaged over to neck and forehead to alleviate the headache; it did wonders for me. A mixture of Panaway, Valor and Peppermint oils diminishes my migraine within half an hour. A gentle rubbing of sinus, temples, neck and forehead can alleviate the pain.

Nothing helped me more than keeping a headache diary. Causes of migraine are unknown but to understand it, a record must made about its recurrence, periodicity and cycle. It helped me comprehend my personal triggers and what I deduced from it was that low blood sugar and lack of sleep prompted migraine. As a result, I don't skip my meals and take proper sleep for 8 hours, which prevented migraine.

Though medication is sometimes necessary, by taking care of one's self, migraine can be prevented and controlled.

Appendix Two: Stress Relieving Advice

Here, one sufferer explains the methods they use to beat stress.

Stress is one of the biggest causes of illness in the United States today. It can lead to cancer, depression, hair loss, migraines and overall poor health. As a migraine sufferer I have realized that a lot of my episodes are caused by stress. I have noticed that during times of great stress caused by work and or family challenges I get major migraine headaches. This has caused me to be more aware of the things that trigger my stress. Below are a few steps that have successfully helped keep my stress level under control.

1. Exercise/Jogging/Yoga- Put on some of your favorite music and go for a Jog, do some aerobics, some Yoga or go for a brisk walk. Do this for a minimum of 30 minutes. After this you will feel refreshed and full of energy.
2. Prayer/Meditation- Some of us believe in speaking to a higher being seeking guidance (prayer) and or Meditation. Through meditation you can analyze the situations that cause you stress. You will be surprise how quick you can come up with a solution. Meditation and prayer help to clear your head and lighten your mental load.
3. Therapy- I know some of us do not believe in speaking to strangers about our problems. However, going to therapy is a great way to relief some stress. Not only does it allow you to speak to a professional about the things you are going through. But, it also gives you the security of knowing that your secrets are safe. Unlike the uncertainties of getting judged by families and friends.
4. Keep a Journal- Jot down all the things that cause you to stress. When does it happen? What triggers it? And how

Appendix Two: Stress Relieving Advice

      can you avoid it. This will give you more insight on how to handle everyday stressors.
5. Diet/Drink tea- Eating more fruits and vegetables will help you balance your hormones. Also drinking tea such as Ginseng, green tea, St. John's worth will help you relax after a long day.
6. Read a book- There are a wide variety of self-help books that will help you manage stress. Some of these are written by people like you and me that have gone through similar experiences. It is always good to know that we are not the only ones that go through certain situations. Makes us feel normal and know that there is a solution to every problem.

There are many causes of stress in our lives. This can cause a great deal of setbacks. Life is too short to allow such things to hinder us from living happy, healthy and successful lives. We must keep stressors in our lives under control by finding ways to minimize them. Practice these steps and find which one works best for you. Also focus on your blessings, all the positive you have in your life. Your children, your health, a great career etc. are just a few of the things we should be thankful for. Waking up every morning is a blessing in itself.

Resources

Forums and Support Groups

It is always useful to talk to patients with similar experiences. People often discover tips quite by accident that they find are helpful for managing their migraines and they are more than happy to share these tips with others.

Likewise, support groups are an excellent way of helping a patient to realise that they are not alone and that there is help available

Inspire.
Inspire.com has a forum for migraine sufferers. People need to sign up to the site before they can contribute. New members are free to discuss their symptoms, join in discussions or start their own.
https://www.inspire.com

WebMD
WebMD has a forum dedicated to migraines. Members of the site offer useful advice and share their experiences of diagnosis, symptoms, effective treatments etc.

It is quite an active site and there is almost always a new discussion and a conversation to contribute to.

Go to www.webmd.com and search for "forum migraines"

Neuro Talk
This forum allows people to post discussions on all topics neurological. Registered members can contribute to other threads or if they have questions, then they can post threads of their own.
http://neurotalk.psychcentral.com

Resources

Healing Well

Healing Well is an online community where migraine sufferers can share their experiences about the different types of medications and managing symptoms.
The site is open to new members and everyone is very welcoming to new members:
http://www.healingwell.com

Finding Support

As well as the forums detailed in the book, there are other ways of getting support and advice. There are several charities and organisations that offer advice packs and tips to help patients manage their migraines better. Here's a list of just some of the organisations that offer help to migraine sufferers.
Migraine Action
Migraine Trust
Headache Australia
Migraine Research Foundation
Another way that is proving increasingly popular is to get in contact with fellow sufferers through social media. Migraine patients often use sites such as Twitter and Facebook to share their experiences and to offer advice and help to other sufferers.

Finding Suppliers

All of the vitamins and herbs detailed in this book are readily available from health stores. If there is any problem sourcing the products locally, then one of the many online stores should be able to supply them
Products like forehead strips and travel sickness bands can be bought from chemists or online from major retailers such as Amazon so if there are difficulties finding any of the products, then this is a good option.

Resources

Clinical Trials

If you are interested in taking part in clinical trials for migraine treatments, these sites list all of the current trials that are open. Studies in the US can be found by going to:
http://www.clinicaltrials.gov

The National Health Service website has links to the current trials being held in the UK. Details can be found at:
http://www.nhs.uk

Further Reading

Migraine and Other Headaches (at your fingertips) Fontebasso, Manuela
The Smart and Easy Guide to Migraine and Headache Relief, Lowery, Sara
50 things you can do today to manage migraines, Green, Wendy
Coping with Headaches and Migraine, Frith, Alison
Heal your Headache, Buchholz, David

Published by IMB Publishing 2014

Copyright and Trademarks. This publication is Copyright 2013 by IMB Publishing. All products, publications, software and services mentioned and recommended in this publication are protected by trademarks. In such instance, all trademarks & copyright belong to the respective owners. All rights reserved. No part of this book may be reproduced or transferred in any form or by any means, graphic, electronic, or mechanical, including photocopying, recording, taping, or by any information storage retrieval system, without the written permission of the author. Pictures used in this book are either royalty free pictures bought from stock-photo websites or have the source mentioned underneath the picture. Disclaimer and Legal Notice. This product is not legal or medical advice and should not be interpreted in that manner. You need to do your own due-diligence to determine if the content of this product is right for you. The author and the affiliates of this product are not liable for any damages or losses associated with the content in this product. While every attempt has been made to verify the information shared in this publication, neither the author nor the affiliates assume any responsibility for errors, omissions or contrary interpretation of the subject matter herein. Any perceived slights to any specific person(s) or organization(s) are purely unintentional. We have no control over the nature, content and availability of the web sites listed in this book. The inclusion of any web site links does not necessarily imply a recommendation or endorse the views expressed within them. IMB Publishing takes no responsibility for, and will not be liable for, the websites being temporarily unavailable or being removed from the internet. The accuracy and completeness of information provided herein and opinions stated herein are not guaranteed or warranted to produce any particular results and the advice and strategies, contained herein may not be suitable for every individual. The author shall not be liable for any loss incurred as a consequence of the use and application, directly or indirectly, of any information presented in this work. This publication is designed to provide information in regards to the subject matter covered. The information included in this book has been compiled to give an overview of ocular migraines and detail some of the symptoms, treatments etc. that are available to people with this condition. It is not intended to give medical advice. For a firm diagnosis of your condition, and for a treatment plan suitable for you, you should consult your doctor or consultant. The writer of this book and the publisher are not responsible for any damages or negative consequences following any of the treatments or methods highlighted in this book. Website links are for informational purposes and should not be seen as a personal endorsement; the same applies to the products detailed in this book. The reader should also be aware that although the web links included were correct at the time of writing, they may become out of date in the future.

CPSIA information can be obtained at www.ICGtesting.com
Printed in the USA
BVOW11s1014190814

363415BV00036B/1674/P